Springer Series: THE TEACHING OF NURSING

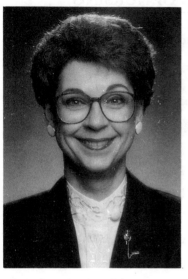

Theresa M. Valiga, EdD, RN, received her bachelor's degree in nursing from Trenton State College and her master's and doctoral degrees, both in Nursing Education, from Teachers College, Columbia University. She has been a faculty member at Trenton State College, Seton Hall University. Georgetown University, and Villanova University, and she currently holds the position of Dean and Professor of the School of Nursing at Fairfield University in Connecticut. Dr. Valiga's primary research interest relates to student cognitive development and critical thinking. Her publications and presentations center around this topic as well as leadership development, creativity in teaching, and various professional issues. She is the author of several articles, has co-authored *The Nurse Educator in Academia: Strategies for Success,* serves on the national boards of Sigma Theta Tau and Phi Kappa Phi, and is a recipient of several awards, including the Sigma Theta Tau International Award for Excellence in Education.

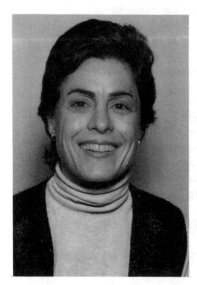

Elizabeth R. Bruderle, MSN, RN, is an Instructor in the College of Nursing at Villanova University. Currently a doctoral candidate at Widener University, she received a master's degree from Villanova University, a bachelor's degree from Neumann College, and a diploma from the Fitzgerald Mercy Hospital School of Nursing. Mrs. Bruderle's research interest focuses on factors that affect how nursing students learn caring. She has co-authored several articles on the use of the arts and humanities to teach nursing concepts, and has taught a graduate course entitled, Creative Teaching Strategies in Nursing Education: Using the Humanities.

Using the Arts and Humanities to Teach Nursing

A Creative Approach

Theresa M. Valiga, EdD, RN
Elizabeth R. Bruderle, MSN, RN

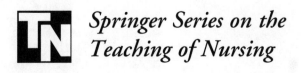

*Springer Series on the
Teaching of Nursing*

Springer Publishing Company, Inc.
536 Broadway
New York, NY 10012-3955

Cover design by Margaret Dunin
Production Editor: Pam Ritzer

97 98 99 00 01 / 5 4 3 2 1

Library of Congress Cataloging-in-Publication Data

Valiga, Theresa M.
   Using the arts and humanities to teach nursing: a creative approach/
Theresa M. Valiga, Elizabeth R. Bruderle.
      p.   cm.
   Includes bibliographical references and index.
   ISBN 0-8261-9420-6
   1. Nursing—Study and teaching.   2. Medicine and the humanities.
I. Bruderle, Elizabeth R. II. Title.
RT73. V346   1997
610.73'071—dc20   96-26797
                                                                          CIP

Printed in the United States of America

This book is dedicated to my husband, Bob, who has supported me throughout this effort and my entire career. His patience, understanding, and encouragement have sustained me through working weekends, tight deadlines, and unexpected pressures, and for that I am ever grateful. The book also is dedicated to the many faculty colleagues and hundreds of students who have shared their ideas and insights, challenged my thinking, and given me the strength to continue to pursue my goal of making nursing education exciting, stimulating, and enjoyable. I think I have learned more from them than from any book I've read or conference I've attended, and I thank them for all they have given me over the years.

— TMV

It is with sincere gratitude that I dedicate this book to my husband, Jerry, and to our children, Stephen, Christopher, and Karen. They provided me with understanding and support and they waited patiently while I completed my work. I also wish to acknowledge my parents; their ongoing encouragement has been a gift.

— ERB

Contents

Contributors

Linda Carman Copel,
Ph.D., R.N., C.S.
Associate Professor
College of Nursing
Villanova University
Villanova, PA 19085-1690

Nancy C. Sharts-Hopko,
Ph.D., R.N., FAAN
Associate Professor
College of Nursing
Villanova University
Villanova, PA 19085-1690

Marycarol McGovern,
Ph.D., R.N.
Assistant Professor
College of Nursing
Villanova University
Villanova, PA 19085-1690

Catherine Todd Magel,
Ed.D., R.N.
Assistant Professor
College of Nursing
Villanova University
Villanova, PA 19085-1690

Foreword

Genevieve M. Bartol, EdD, RN

Nursing education draws knowledge from many disciplines. The sciences, humanities, and even the arts are considered important components of nursing curricula. Scientific breakthroughs and rapidly expanding technology, however, have granted the sciences a certain ascendancy. The sheer mass of information that nurses are expected to assimilate further threatens the liberal education that nurses value.

Scientific skill and technological proficiency are not sufficient for quality nursing. The criticism and skepticism of a scientific stance by itself tends to question the validity of all meanings. Depersonalization and fragmentation of life results from extreme specialization in a complex technological environment. Nurses need to see the essence of human life in its scientific and humanistic aspects. An integrated outlook is important because individuals are organic totalities and not just a composite of separate parts. Scientific knowledge must be informed with wisdom, and technological skill must be tempered with tenderness. We need nursing practitioners with a dual sensibility; possessing scientific and technological expertise and alive to humanistic disciplines.

Moreover, courses are too often taught as separate entities with no reference to the subject matter of other courses in the curriculum. Students go from one course to another without understanding how the knowledge and skills they accumulate relate to nursing. Generally, they take the curriculum as it is presented, a traditional sequence of separate elements. Few students appreciate or understand the comprehensive pattern of the whole curriculum in which the various elements are located. It is difficult to grasp a sense of the whole with such a compartmentalized approach.

Readers of this book will be reminded of the significance of the humanities and arts for nursing and find help for reintegrating them into nursing courses. Each discipline represents different approaches to truth; none have a monopoly of knowledge. Knowledge from the sciences is vital for nursing practice. But the arts and humanities elucidate particular aspects of what human beings are and offer a powerful focus for transformative learning experiences. In their book Valiga and Bruderle remind us of our values and provide us with a guide for reintegrating the arts and humanities into nursing education.

It is difficult to maintain a humanistic orientation amidst a rapidly changing health care system. Greater acuity in highly specialized inpatient care settings along with a radical shift to community-based care and managed care present us with new challenges. The arts and humanities, which are concerned with human thought and relationships, can provide us with insights that should not be ignored.

Genevieve M. Bartol, EdD, RN
Professor
The University of North Carolina at Greensboro
School of Nursing
Greensboro, North Carolina

Preface

Nursing education currently is witnessing an emphasis on the development of critical thinking skills, a call for greater creativity and innovation in teaching, suggestions for a curriculum revolution, and an acknowledgment of the significance of the liberal education component of higher education. In light of such trends, nurse educators are exploring new ways to enhance the learning of their students that involve both the learner and the teacher. The integration of the arts and humanities into the teaching of nursing is a legitimate way to achieve such goals.

Despite the unlimited possibilities for and potential benefits of integrating the arts and humanities into the teaching of nursing, there is very little in the literature that addresses this approach in any great detail. Some articles have been written that speak to the benefits of using the humanities to enhance learning and to individual experiences with a humanities-related assignment (Bartol, 1989; Darbyshire, 1995; Germain, 1986; Hoshiko, 1985; Murray & Copeland, 1992; Peck, 1993; Peden & Staten, 1994; Vande Zande, 1995; Younger, 1990; Young–Mason, 1988). In addition, one anthology (Styles & Moccia, 1993) offers examples of writings that relate to nursing or aspects of nursing practice, and a recent book (Chinn & Watson, 1994) explores art and aesthetics in nursing.

Despite this progress, many of the works published in this arena are narrow in scope and limited in the examples offered; thus, they may not be particularly useful to faculty who do not teach the concepts/content described in the work or who teach a different level of students. Additionally, the published texts that relate to this creative approach to teaching do not address how these items can be used to help neophytes learn nursing.

In essence, then, no comprehensive source exists for faculty, and there is a gap in the literature. This book is designed to fill that gap and offer nurse educators a wide variety of specific examples of how the arts and humanities—through their varied media—can become an integral part of the teaching of nursing.

This book has been designed primarily for those educators who have responsibility for teaching nursing, either to students of nursing or to practicing nurses. It can be used by the faculty in any nursing education program (graduate, baccalaureate, associate degree, diploma, or licensed practical nurse), and by staff development educators as well. In addition, the book can serve as a text for graduate students enrolled in teaching strategy courses or in programs preparing educators.

In writing this book, the authors have drawn on their experiences teaching a graduate-level elective course entitled, "Creative Teaching Strategies in Nursing: Using the Humanities," which has been taught at Villanova University's College of Nursing since 1985. They also have drawn on a continuing education workshop they presented on this topic and a video production (with related student and teacher guides) entitled, "Nursing: Artistic Expressions," which they have developed and used to introduce beginning undergraduate students to the profession. Finally, the ideas in this book have evolved from a chapter written by the authors in Chinn and Watson's *Art & Aesthetics in Nursing* (Bruderle & Valiga, 1994) and a research study they completed (Valiga & Bruderle, 1994) that explored the concepts integral to nursing education programs.

The book has been organized to provide an overview of the arts and humanities in terms of their goals and purposes. A variety of art forms—novels, short stories, children's literature, poetry, films, television, music, sculpture, paintings, opera, photography, and drama—are explored along with the advantages, disadvantages, and sources of each.

Following this general introduction to the arts and humanities and the overview of specific art forms, selected concepts that are common in nursing education and practice are examined. An analysis of each concept is undertaken to establish a common basis and a foundation for the kind of understandings we hope students will achieve related to the concept. Each of the chapters concludes with a variety of specific examples of how the arts and humanities can be used to help students learn the concept.

Our readers are invited to be open to the possibilities that await them when they allow themselves to be creative and to think in new ways. The arts and humanities resources that can be used to enhance learning in nursing are unlimited, and they certainly can make teaching and learning more fun and more productive. So, sit back, allow yourself to consider the ideas offered here, and enjoy!

REFERENCES

Bartol, G. (1989). Creative literature: An aid to nursing practice. *Nursing & Health Care, 10,* 453–457.

Bruderle, E. R., & Valiga, T. M. (1994). In P. L. Chinn & J. Watson (Eds.), *Art & aesthetics in nursing* (pp.117–144). New York: National League for Nursing.

Chinn, P., & Watson, J. (1994). *Art & aesthetics in nursing.* New York: National League for Nursing.

Darbyshire, P. (1995). Lessons from literature: Caring, interpretation, and dialogue. *Journal of Nursing Education, 34,* 211–215.

Germain, C. P. (1986). Using literature to teach nursing. *Journal of Nursing Education, 25*(2), 84–86.

Hoshiko, B. R. (1985). Nursing diagnosis at the art museum. *Nursing Outlook, 33*(1), 32–36.

Murray, B. L., & Copeland, L. G. (1992). Is there a place for Phil Donahue in the classroom? *Journal of Nursing Education, 31*(6), 285–286.

Peck, S. E. (1993). Monitoring student learning with poetry. *Journal of Nursing Education, 32*(4), 190–191.

Peden, A., & Staten, R. (1994). The use of the humanities in psychiatric nursing education. *Journal of Nursing Education, 33,* 41–42.

Styles, M. M., & Moccia, P. (1993). *On nursing: A literary celebration. An anthology.* New York: National League for Nursing.

Valiga, T. M., & Bruderle, E. R. (1994). Concepts included in and critical to nursing curricula: An analysis. *Journal of Nursing Education, 33,* 118–124.

Vande Zande, G. (1995). The liberal arts and professional nursing: Making the connections. *Journal of Nursing Education, 34*(2), 93–94.

Younger, J. (1990). Literary works as a mode of knowing. *Image: Journal of Nursing Scholarship, 22,* 39–42.

Young–Mason, J. (1988). Literature as a mirror to compassion. *Journal of Professional Nursing, 4,* 299–301.

Aknowledgments

This book could not have been completed without the outstanding contributions of our Villanova University College of Nursing faculty colleagues, Dr. Linda Copel, Dr. Nancy Sharts-Hopko, Dr. Marycarol McGovern, and Dr. Cathy Todd Magel. The chapters they prepared for this book reflect their expertise, their openness to creative thinking, and their willingness to engage in collegial collaboration.

We also want to acknowledge and thank the many students who have enrolled in the graduate-level elective course on "Creative Teaching Strategies in Nursing: Using the Humanities" since it was initiated at Villanova University in 1985. These students completed innovative, exciting projects that demonstrate the ways in which the arts and humanities can be used to teach nursing, and many have gone on to incorporate these and other ideas into their own teaching with undergraduate students, as well as staff nurses in clinical agencies. Their creativity, enthusiasm, and willingness to take on the challenge of "being different" stimulated us to continue to pursue our interest in integrating the arts and humanities into nursing education and write this book.

Finally, we wish to recognize the students we have had in a variety of classes where the arts and humanities have been used as strategies to facilitate learning. These undergraduate and graduate students have tolerated our "craziness" in asking them to read poems or novels, watch television shows and movies, or write stories, all in the name of "learning nursing." They have been a joy to know, and they have helped us grow and continue to be open to new ideas and possibilities.

TMV
ERB

Part I

UNDERSTANDING THE PLACE OF THE HUMANITIES IN NURSING EDUCATION

1

The Arts and Humanities: Their Relevance to Nursing Education

Nursing is an art; and if it is to be made an art,
it requires as exclusive a devotion, as hard a
            preparation, as any painter's or sculptor's work;
for what is the having to do with dead canvas or cold
            marble,
compared with having to do with the living body—
            the temple of God's spirit?
It is one of the Fine Arts;
I had almost said, the finest of the Fine Arts.

— *Florence Nightingale*

Nursing practice today takes place in an arena that is challenging, ever-changing, complex, and characterized by increasing specialization and a heightened use of myriad technologies. Professional nurses who practice in this environment must be flexible, adaptable, technologically proficient, and have a sound scientific foundation. Perhaps more importantly, however, professional nurses must maintain their commitment to humanistic health care, which has been identified as the uniqueness of nursing (Donaldson, 1983). Indeed, "without the humanistic perspective, the uniqueness of the nursing discipline becomes lost" (Vande Zande, 1995, p. 93).

But just what is a humanistic perspective? Nurses who maintain their commitment to humanistic health care convey a caring attitude, attend to the concerns and feelings of others, and are sensitive to the contexts in which others live, their cultures, and the unique ways they live in the world. It is when they interact with people who are experiencing critical junctures in their lives that nurses most need to express and maintain their commitment to humanistic care, for it is at such times that humanistic care is needed most.

3

THE DOMAINS OF LEARNING

The work of nursing is intellectually, physically, and emotionally demanding, and nurse educators, who are helping students prepare for such a role, must attend to all three domains of learning if they are to graduate competent, humanistic nurses. Typically, our academic programs focus on learning in the *cognitive domain*, where the emphasis is on knowledge acquisition, the transfer of information, understanding, application, and evaluation. We measure learning in this domain through tests, term papers, class presentations, case studies, nursing care plans, participation in discussions, or completion of projects.

Because of the nature of nursing practice, our educational programs also attend carefully to learning in the *psychomotor domain*, which focuses on manipulation skills, efficiency, accuracy, and competence with technologies. Learning in this area is measured by students' performance in the clinical area or the learning laboratory.

The emotional or *affective domain*, however, typically receives very little attention in nursing education. The affective domain deals with beliefs, values, and attitudes, which are more abstract, less tangible, and more difficult to measure than are outcomes in the other two domains. Faculty may argue that (a) learning objectives in the affective domain are inappropriate ones for higher education because values are formed when we are children rather than adults, (b) faculty should not be involved in "indoctrination," and (c) measuring the achievement of such objectives is totally subjective and, therefore, should not be done. As a result of these and other arguments, faculty sometimes abandon the affective domain in favor of the cognitive or psychomotor areas. However, if the aim of higher education is the total development of the student (Kohlberg & Mayer, 1972), an aim that is evident in the philosophy, mission, or outcomes of many nursing programs, nursing faculty do students a disservice when they fail to give as much emphasis to the affective domain as they do to the other two areas.

As is the case with other faculty, nursing faculty have become "addict[ed] to coverage" (Paul, 1994, p. 11) and see their primary responsibility as covering content, thus emphasizing learning in the cognitive domain. As a result, our courses and approaches to teaching frequently emphasize remembering rather than understanding, and answering rather than thoughtfully responding. The result of these kinds of learning experiences in didactic-oriented courses is that "students develop the illusion of understanding many things that they, in fact, don't really understand at all" (Paul, 1994, p. 1). When faculty engage in "what John Goodlad has called 'frontal teaching' . . . cram[ming] facts and information into students' heads and not giving them enough time to understand what they are learning" (Hanford, 1994, p. 6), they do not develop critical thinkers or enhance humanistic perspectives.

CRITICAL THINKING

Although a case has just been made to increase our emphasis on the affective domain, nurse educators cannot do that to the exclusion of focusing on cognitive, or thinking, skills. Indeed, a healthy balance must be achieved. But as one reflects on the nature of critical thinking, one realizes that it is not a matter of "either/or," a position supported by Woditsch, Schlesinger and Giardina (1987). Instead, nursing education must attend to cognitive, or thinking, skills and affective, or humanistic, perspectives, and the use of the arts and humanities can facilitate that dual focus.

Critical thinking has been defined as "reflective and reasonable thinking that is focused on deciding what to believe or what to do" (Ennis, 1985, p. 45). It is thinking that is guided by reason, or responsible thinking that is sensitive to context and that can be judged by others in light of standards and expectations. Critical thinking also has been thought of as purposeful and goal-directed thinking.

Whatever particular definition of critical thinking one might prefer, there are several elements that characterize critical thinking, and each can be developed through the use of the arts and humanities. One of those elements relates to *knowing clearly just what the problem at hand is*, describing its components, conceptualizing it from different points of view, taking the complex whole of the problem into account, and examining issues rationally, logically, and coherently. Listening to the message conveyed in Phil Collins' song, "Just Another Day in Paradise," can help students crystallize the problem of alienation in our society—alienation of the poor, the homeless, the elderly—and appreciate its complexity.

Another very important element of critical thinking (Brookfield,

1987) has to do with *examining the assumptions* that underlie what people say and do. Critical thinkers look at the basic beliefs they have about themselves, others, and people in general, and they do not stereotype, jump to conclusions, or act without thinking. Robert Frost's poem, "The Road Not Taken," deals with making decisions, and decisions are based on the kind of information we have at hand, the assumptions we make about the potential outcomes of our choices, what we think others would want us to do, our personal strengths and weaknesses, and so on. Thus, use of this poem can enhance critical thinking as well as heighten students' insights and understandings about people.

Critical thinking also involves *envisioning possible solutions* to problems, generating ideas, reflecting on possibilities, and conceiving alternate courses of action. In addition, critical thinkers *exercise sound argument skills* when considering options and various viewpoints. They can detect fallacies in reasoning, evaluate the quality and relevance of conclusions drawn or the inferences made from data, consider possible contradictions, separate relevant from irrelevant data, and weigh the accuracy and logic of evidence. They also raise relevant questions and critique solutions as a way to see that the best course of action is taken. The 1981 film, *Whose Life Is It Anyway?*, offers an excellent example of how decisions get made for patients. It sensitizes the viewer not only to the physical struggles of a young man who is paralyzed but also to his emotional struggles and his need to examine alternate solutions to problems.

Critical thinkers tend to *use higher order cognitive processes and intellectual skills*. They can logically organize knowledge from various sources, even though much of it may be conflicting. They view knowledge as temporary and are comfortable solving problems, even when there is a great deal of uncertainty and unpredictability in situations. Viewing any abstract painting by Picasso forces one to deal with the unexpected; for example, a painting of a woman may depict an upside-down head, two noses, and a breast where an arm ought to be. Such a painting could be used to help students think about how they can make sense of conflicting information and respond to situations that are unpredictable.

Making judgments, particularly in complex situations and particularly on the basis of sound reason and adequate evidence, is another element of critical thinking. This involves drawing valid conclusions and making correct inferences. Students might be asked to think about what is really meant by the poems in the book, *When I Am an Old Woman, I Shall Wear Purple* (Martz, 1987). After reading these poems, faculty could help students explore the inferences or conclusions they draw about living, aging, and facing the end of one's life.

One of the most significant components of critical thinking is *having a questioning attitude.* Critical thinkers engage in activities with reflective, informed, healthy skepticism. In other words, they consistently raise relevant questions, play with ideas, maintain an attitude of openness, and display intellectual curiosity. They are disposed to think carefully about issues and situations, constantly ask questions, and have a critical spirit. The use of art in general, with its openness to interpretation and its personal nature, can serve to promote a questioning attitude. When one student looks at "The Pietà" and sees compassion, another sees grief, and yet another sees hope, faculty can use these interpretations to initiate a discussion of why different people focus on or "see" different things in the same situation. They also could guide students in a discussion of how our culture and religious orientation influence our view of the world, and why experiences have different degrees of meaning to us throughout our lives. All of this helps students appreciate that asking questions is a healthy way to approach the world and, indeed, a necessary skill to have if nurses are to provide quality care to patients and families.

Finally, critical thinking involves *evaluating one's own thinking,* reflecting on one's actions, and being creative. And critical thinkers are characterized by *caring passionately about what they study and what they do.* Asking students to watch a television show that presents a negative depiction of nurses (e.g., *Nightingales* or *General Hospital*) could be an impetus for them to consider how deeply they feel about the public's perceptions of nursing, and it could even stimulate them to take action in relation to such passions. Indeed, as Stevens (1995) said, if students are to be prepared to be responsible professionals, they must develop a sense of passion. And "passion is sparked by exciting the student to the possibilities of the profession and of health care. It is fostered with a humanistic approach to teaching—one that emphasizes development of 'selfhood' as well as clinical and scientific expertise" (Stevens, 1995, p. 99). The arts and humanities to which students are exposed within the context of their nursing courses can be the spark that ignites such passion.

Critical thinking, obviously, is much more than problem solving, decision making, or using the nursing process. It also is more than merely a cognitive exercise. Indeed, without critical thinking, college may be thought of merely as an exercise in endurance rather than the experience in education educators hope it will be. If one concurs that the true benefits of education are the personal insights and thought processes that result from the study of a discipline, rather than the facts and information accumulated, then critical thinking is a vital skill to be developed, particularly in nursing students who will be practicing in a world characterized by diversity, uncertainty, and ambiguity.

Students who are critical thinkers have been personally transformed (Chaffee, 1994), and students who have been assisted to develop in the affective domain, as well as in the cognitive and psychomotor areas, also undergo a personal transformation. Such students have a greater sense of self-knowledge, achieve a clearer understanding of the separateness and individuality of others, and are better able to integrate and connect the experiences of others within themselves (Wilson, 1974). Nurses who are to practice in the health care world of the 21st century—with its ambiguity, need to make decisions in uncertainty, unpredictability, infinite possibilities, explosive change, and rapidly expanding knowledge—must be prepared in all three domains, and nurse educators must take responsibility to provide for this kind of preparation.

But how can faculty develop students as critical thinkers and facilitate the integration of the science of nursing with the art of nursing? Perhaps one answer lies in the use of the arts and humanities.

INTEGRATION OF LIBERAL EDUCATION AND NURSING

Few would argue that the educational preparation of a professional nurse needs to include learning in the arts and humanities. In fact, the National League for Nursing's Baccalaureate and Higher Degree Council includes among its criteria for accreditation the requirement that the baccalaureate curriculum be "supported by cognates in the arts, sciences and humanities" (National League for Nursing, 1991, p. 20), and the American Association of Colleges of Nursing (1986) stressed the need for nurses to have a liberal education and for nursing faculty to integrate knowledge from the liberal arts and sciences into nursing education.

In light of this requirement and philosophical beliefs that learning in the arts and humanities is essential to prepare a truly educated person, undergraduate nursing curricula incorporate courses in literature, philosophy, history, religion, theology, and the arts. One must question, however, the ways in which insights gained from courses in these fields are built upon, drawn upon, or integrated into nursing courses, which typically are taken in the upper division after the arts and humanities courses are completed. In other words, "the question is not *whether* nurses need a healthy mix of professional and liberal learning, but *how* the blend might best be achieved" (Newell, 1985, p. 253). If higher education is to assist students to develop as holistic human beings, the integration of the arts and humanities with nursing cannot be ignored, lest each be seen as isolated experiences that have little or nothing in common. Yet this is what seems to happen.

In a study of registered nurses' perception of liberal education, Hagerty and Early (1993) reported that nurses had acknowledged the benefits of a liberal education: expanding their minds, exposing them to different perspectives and ideas, helping them appreciate a larger world, enhancing their self-awareness, and promoting their receptivity to the world. However, despite these benefits, many of these nurses admitted that they were "unable to see the relevance of their liberal arts and science courses *while in school* [emphasis added] and only came to appreciate content and perspectives after additional life and work experiences" (p. 154).

Similar findings were reported by Peck and Jennings (1989) who found that the 91 senior baccalaureate students and alumnae they studied generally thought that the liberal arts and humanities were an important aspect of their educational experience. Interestingly, however, the subjects in this study believed that *they themselves* were the ones to make the links between liberal arts and nursing; nursing faculty were reported not to have helped in making those connections. While we might be encouraged by the finding that students and alumnae valued the liberal arts in their preparation as nurses, we must be cautious in that enthusiasm for two reasons. First, instead of defining liberal arts in terms of philosophy, literature, religion, history, and the fine arts, as they typically are defined in the literature, these researchers apparently defined liberal arts as including biology, chemistry, English, nutrition, psychology, and sociology (p. 410), subjects one would expect students to see as relevant to nursing. In addition, the finding that faculty were not particularly influential in helping students interrelate nursing and the arts and humanities leads one to question the views of faculty regarding the liberal arts: Are the arts and humanities truly valued by nursing faculty? And do nursing faculty themselves see the "links" between the arts and humanities and nursing?

A more recent study (Zaborowska, 1995) examined senior baccalaureate nursing students' self-reported involvement in activities related to liberal education goals. It included 201 students from 11 programs in the Midwest who were asked how they spent their time, the nature and quality of their activities, and the gains they believed they made during college. The researcher found that students spent significantly more time on academic activities (e.g., library work) than they did on liberal arts activities, such as art, music, and theater. Subjects also believed they made the least amount of progress in meeting educational goals related to understanding and enjoying art, music, and drama. These results, notes the researcher, "validate the concerns stated in many of the recent national reports about the narrow experience many students have in college" (p. 160).

Perhaps nurse educators need to focus more on integrating the arts and humanities *into nursing courses,* so that students can be helped to see the relationship between the two areas while they are learning about their profession, and can be better prepared to face the many challenges provided by professional nursing practice. In other words, education must focus as much on the development of the nurse as a person as on the development of a knowledge base and skills. The professional nurse who can combine the science of nursing with the art of nursing and the humanistic perspective developed through a study of the liberal arts, may be better prepared to engage in such a challenging practice role.

A quarter of a century ago, Dickoff and James (1970) and Priest (1970) noted that the education of nurses incorporates preparing them for their profession *and* educating them as human beings living in a world of diverse people. In light of this goal, these authors acknowledged the importance of the humanities in the educational process because the humanities address the responses of human beings to a variety of experiences. Thus, nursing faculty have a responsibility to attend to the integration of nursing with the arts and humanities.

Students need to learn to *blend* liberal arts and professional values and abilities, and the two need to "depend on each other" (Armour & Fuhrmann, 1989, p. 2). Indeed, faculty need to address and resolve the "ancient dichotomy that has plagued American higher education at least since the founding of the land grant colleges" (Curtis, 1985, p. 10), namely, the dichotomy between liberal and professional education.

Perhaps blending the liberal arts and nursing—making "greater use of humanities, arts, and social science content *in nursing courses*" [emphasis added] (Newell, 1989, p. 69) rather than "'parceling out' chunks of the curriculum" (Newell, 1989, p. 69) to various disciplines— is one way to achieve critical thinking and affective domain goals. To paraphrase Nietzsche, "A teacher is an artist with concepts" (Chaffee, 1994, p. 25); the arts and humanities may help nursing faculty be more creative "artists" in the educational process.

Lee (1986, p. 62) asserted that "the art and craft of teaching requires that one has a repertoire of teaching moves and is skilled in their use, but more important, that one is able to draw on educational imagination and invent new moves that advance the students from one place to another along the intellectual path." The integration of the arts and humanities *into nursing courses* is a "new move" for most nurse educators, but the benefits of using the humanities may help educators prepare the kind of nurses needed to practice in our complex, technological, ever-changing health care environment.

WHY THE ARTS AND HUMANITIES?

The word humanities comes from the Latin for humanity. The humanities, therefore, may be thought of as that branch of knowledge which deals with what it means to be human, to live authentically, and to share with others. They strive to "preserve as much as possible of the variety, the uniqueness, the unexpectedness, the complexity, the originality" (Crane, 1967, p. 12) of individual human beings.

The humanities provide for a liberal education and include the disciplines of philosophy, literature, history, languages, religion, architecture, and the fine arts, which in turn include music, paintings, sculpture, drama, and dance. However, they have been looked upon, "during most of the modern period, as means to the realization of some larger ideal or use over and above the understanding and appreciation of . . . specific subject matter" (Crane, 1967, p. 5); thus, they tend to achieve affective domain goals more so than cognitive ones. In light of this higher order goal, we must remember that liberal education "is not the exclusive province of any set of academic departments or administrative divisions" (Newell, 1989, p. 69). Nurse educators, therefore, can legitimately use the arts and humanities as part of their teaching repertoire *within existing courses.*

If educators are to help nursing students learn what it means to be human, they must guide students to examine their attitudes toward life, the place of the individual in society, the nature of our common humanity, the significance of human endeavors, and the relationships and responsibilities of individuals to one another. There must be a focus on people, their experiences, their response to and interpretation of the world around them, and the meanings they make.

The humanities provide such a focus and a forum for this kind of examination. In addition, they allow and encourage unique interpretations of events and situations, acknowledge the importance of feelings in our lives, focus on people and what they experience, provide opportunities for individuals to confront and deal with uncertainty, and promote individuality.

Many individuals view the arts and humanities merely as "a fine veneer that enables [us] to communicate socially with others and provides an interesting diversion to manage stress" (Bartol, 1986, p. 21). In addition, the arts and humanities often are seen as doing little more than providing trivial knowledge that may be useful at cocktail parties or in some game, such as *Jeopardy!* And nursing students often think of the humanities merely as courses that must be endured in order to earn a baccalaureate degree. But the humanities are much more.

"A liberal arts education in our society is generally thought to enrich our lives, to provide breadth and understanding, to teach us something, to enhance intellectual vision and to be the basis upon which we gain knowledge" (Franke, 1986, p. 3). By exposing us to creative products, a diverse world, and the many interpretations of that world, the humanities help us avoid routine. They open us up to new possibilities and new perspectives, and in so doing, they introduce the mysterious and the unknown into our lives, stretch our imaginations, release our capacity for imagination, and liberate the full potential in each of us.

As we reflect on the meaning of a poem or a painting, or as we literally spend days with a character while reading a novel, we often become more aware of our personal values and question them or develop a deeper and longer-lasting commitment to them. The arts and humanities can awaken or elucidate our beliefs and values and help us clarify the personal values that guide our actions. They help us, therefore, to enhance our self-knowledge.

When a character in a film or short story faces a personal dilemma, our own sense of choice and decision is heightened. We are exposed to broader choices and more options, develop new insights into problem solving, decision making, and the resolution of personal conflicts, and we confront larger social issues that "provide contexts for the decisions we must make as a people by raising questions of social purpose" (Text of Cheney's *Report to the President*, 1988, p. A17).

Since the arts and humanities can "take us back in time," they serve to provide an historical context and connections with and insights to the past. In addition, they "enlarge [our] understanding by showing us we are not the first generation to grapple with moral dilemmas" (Text of Cheney's *Report to the President*, 1988, p. A17). In essence, this kind of exposure helps us understand time, processes, and change in ways we might not have understood them before. It also helps us understand the cultural and historical context in which we live and in which nursing is practiced.

The arts and humanities also "convey how the ideas and ideals of our civilization have evolved, thus providing a basis for understanding other cultures" (Text of Cheney's *Report to the President*, 1988, p. A18). They help us grasp the state of the world in which we live and act, and accentuate the multifaceted nature of the world.

Music, drama, paintings, novels, poems, film, and other art forms can expose or sensitize us to certain realities and increase our social consciousness. The shared values that bind people together as a society and the relationships between people and groups can be highlighted, and images of human reality and possibility that increase our sensitivity and our sense of compassion and empathy can be provided.

Since the arts provide opportunities for private moments and reflection, they provide a stimulus for each of us to come to know ourselves and the world around us in very different ways. They inspire us, help liberate our potential, and promote intellectual, cultural, and personal growth, thereby developing the whole person. Indeed, they "provide a framework for lifelong learning about ourselves and the world in which we live" (Text of Cheney's *Report to the President*, 1988, p. A18).

By exposing us to new ideas, new perspectives and new areas of knowledge and understanding, the arts and humanities work to "free the mind from ignorance, prejudice, and slavish dependence on other minds" (Newell, 1989, p. 69). They encourage the expression of original ideas and personal perspectives and thereby help promote differences of opinion and points of view and support an acceptance of such differences.

Perhaps the most significant area affected by exposure to the arts and humanities is the development of the individual himself or herself. Art conveys human qualities and promotes "a heightening of sensory awareness and emotional responsiveness" (Rogers, 1969, p. 12). Art, literature, history, and so on heighten our perceptions and feelings, help us develop greater insights about ourselves and about others, and call upon and develop right-brain skills, thereby stimulating our creativity. They acknowledge the legitimacy of intuitive thinking, and they help us to appreciate and manage the diversity, ambiguity, complexity, and uncertainty that characterize our world. Indeed, "liberal education provides a foundation for understanding human wholeness, human potential, and the complexity of human experiences that influence health" (Reed, 1987, p. 37).

The arts and humanities promote synthesis rather than reductionism. They help us avoid simplification of what is "distinctively human about human achievements" (Booth, 1967, p. xv). The humanities foster the development of an inquiring mind, and "help [us] understand [our]selves in historical, cultural and aesthetic terms" (Arts, Education and Americans Panel, cited in Lee,

1986, p. 62). Mere exposure to the arts themselves initiates us into the artistic, aesthetic domain without trying to make artists or poets out of us, thereby broadening our perspective and understanding. Finally, the arts and humanities "waken us from the numbness that all too frequently accompanies routine" (Bartol, 1986, p. 23). As noted by Hoffman (1939), "the powers of the human mind are infinitely more diverse and profound than we realize. [However], most of us are mentally lazy [and] we miss worlds of experience, as a result of this" (p. 75). Art can awaken the mind by keeping us from growing indifferent and failing to truly see the things that surround us.

The challenges to nurse educators are enormous, but the arts and humanities can be helpful in meeting many of those challenges. As Carr (1994, p. B2) notes, "Teaching is the most difficult task a human being can do because it involves changing the lives of strangers by touching their thoughts and experiences." "Education [needs] to change society rather than maintain the status quo" (Horton, 1990, p. xix), and teachers need to attend to where students are and where they can be, "forever pushing, making them uncomfortable, stretching their minds, helping them grow in their understandings and critical consciousness" (Horton, 1990, p. xx). As teachers, we need to create tasks and learning experiences that "require critical thinking, caring design, deep perplexity, [and] unyielding ambiguity" (Carr, 1994, p. B2) if we are to prepare our students for effective practice in the 21st century. Integrating the arts and humanities into nursing education can provide students with such tasks and learning experiences.

Parr (1982) cited research that documents how today's students are "morally apathetic, now-oriented, and alienated from learning" (p. xiii). He suggested that to reverse this trend, all courses routinely and seriously must incorporate a focus on morals and values, discourage oversimplification, and emphasize critical analysis and informed choice. Parr provided extensive examples of the use of literature as a means to focus on morals and values, but nurse educators need not limit themselves to the medium of literature to facilitate our students' development. By integrating a variety of art forms *with nursing* and *in nursing courses and learning experiences,* nurse educators can find ways to meet this challenge and design learning experiences that yield positive outcomes.

CONCLUSION

Today's nursing students must be prepared to deal with the complexity, ambiguity, uncertainty, and unparalleled change that characterize our world. That world is inhabited by billions of very unique individuals, and graduates of our programs must be prepared to address that uniqueness. In light of the many positive outcomes of "connecting" with the arts and humanities, students of nursing must be exposed to the arts and humanities in significant ways, not only through courses taught by experts in the fields of literature, fine arts, and philosophy, but in nursing courses as well.

Nursing faculty are expected to facilitate the preparation of safe, competent practitioners who provide compassionate care. The elements of safety and competence typically are addressed quite well through the sciences and the current approaches to teaching nursing, but the elements of care and compassion need to be addressed through other means. Faculty can foster a caring attitude through personal and professional role modeling of caring behaviors and a genuine sensitivity to the uniqueness of others. The use of creative teaching strategies, including integrating the arts and humanities into nursing education, also can foster caring and compassion by helping students understand who they are, what it means to be human, and how it feels to care.

"Participatory involvement with the many forms of art does enable us, at the very least, to *see* more in our experience, to *hear* more on normally unheard frequencies, to *become conscious* of what daily routines, habits, and conventions have obscured" (Greene, 1995, 379). In light of these potentials, nurse educators need to help students do more than merely tolerate the liberal arts courses in the curriculum or merely observe "dead canvas or cold marble" (Nightingale, as cited in Donohue, 1985, p. 469). Instead, by integrating the arts and humanities into the teaching and learning experiences they design, faculty can enhance students' appreciation of the intensity of life, the diversity of their fellow human beings, and the richness of the world around them. One does not need to be an expert in literature, sculpture, music, poetry, or drama to use them as tools to facilitate the learning of nursing concepts. What one *does* need, however, is an openness of mind, an appreciation of the art of nursing as well as the science, and a willingness to take risks and use new approaches to stimulate learning and a love of nursing.

REFERENCES

American Association of Colleges of Nursing. (1986). *Essentials of college and university education for professional nursing: Final report.* Washington, DC: Author.

Armour, R. A., & Fuhrmann, B. S. (Eds.). (1989). *Integrating liberal learning and professional education* (New Directions for Teaching and Learning, No. 40). San Francisco: Jossey–Bass.

Bartol, G. M. (1986). Using the humanities in nursing education. *Nurse Educator, 11*(1), 21–23.

Booth, W. C. (1967). Introduction. In R. S. Crane, *The idea of the humanities and other essays: Critical and historical. Volume I* (pp. xiii–xxii). Chicago: University of Chicago Press.

Brookfield, S. (1987). *Developing critical thinking.* San Francisco: Jossey–Bass.

Carr, D. (1994). The lives of learners. *Chronicle of Higher Education, 40*(33), B2.

Chaffee, J. (1994). Teaching for critical thinking. *Educational Vision, 2*(1), 24–25.

Crane, R. S. (1967). *The idea of the humanities and other essays: Critical and historical. Volume I.* Chicago: University of Chicago Press.

Curtis, M. H. (1985). Confronting an ancient dichotomy: A proposal for integrating liberal and professional education. *National Forum, 65*(3), 10–12.

Dickoff, J., & James, P. (1970). Beliefs and values: Bases for curriculum design. *Nursing Research, 19*(5), 415–426.

Donahue, M. P. (1985). *Nursing: The finest art. An illustrated history.* St. Louis: Mosby.

Donaldson, S. (1983). Let us not abandon the humanities. *Nursing Outlook, 31*(1), 40–43.

Ennis, R. H. (1985). A logical basis for measuring critical thinking skills. *Educational Leadership, 43*(2), 44–48.

Franke, R. J. (1986). *Education: For employment or for life.* Chicago: John Nuveen & Co.

Greene, M. (1995). Art and imagination: Reclaiming the sense of possibility. *Phi Delta Kappan, 76*(5), 378–381.

Hagerty, B., & Early, S. L. (1993). Registered nurses' perceptions of liberal education. *Journal of Nursing Education, 32*(4), 151–155.

Hanford, G. (1994). The danger of fragmentation. *Educational Vision, 2*(1), 6–7.

Hoffman, M. (1939). *Sculpture inside and out.* New York: Bonanza Books.

Horton, M. (1990). *The long haul: An autobiography.* New York: Doubleday.

Kohlberg, L., & Mayer, R. (1972). Development as the aim of education. *Harvard Educational Review, 42*(4), 449–496.

Lee, R. T. (1986). The role of the arts in teaching effectively. *Educational Horizons, 64*(2), 62–66.

Martz, S. H. (Ed.) (1987). *When I am an old woman, I shall wear purple.* Watsonville, CA: Papier–Mache Press.

National League for Nursing. (1991). *Criteria and guidelines for the evaluation of baccalaureate and higher degree programs in nursing.* New York: Author.

Newell, L. J. (1985). Shall the twain meet? Liberal education and nursing education (Editorial). *Journal of Professional Nursing, 1*(5), 253–254.

Newell, L. J. (1989). The healing arts and the liberal arts in concert. In R. A. Armour & B. S. Fuhrmann (Eds.), *Integrating liberal learning and professional education* (New Directions for Teaching and Learning, No. 40) (pp. 67–76). San Francisco: Jossey–Bass.

Parr, S. R. (1982). *The moral of the story: Literature, values, and American education.* New York: Teachers College Press.

Paul, R. (1994). Overcoming the addiction to coverage. *Educational Vision, 2*(1), 11.

Peck, M. L., & Jennings, S. (1989). Student perceptions of the links between nursing and the liberal arts. *Journal of Nursing Education, 28*(9), 406–414.

Priest, R. R. (1970). The humanities in the nursing curriculum. In M. Q. Innis (Ed.), *Nursing education in a changing society* (pp. 184–189). Toronto: University of Toronto Press.

Reed, P. G. (1987). Liberal arts and professional nursing education: Integrating knowledge and wisdom. *Nurse Educator, 12*(4), 37–40.

Rogers, L. R. (1969). *The appreciation of the arts/2: Sculpture.* London: Oxford University Press.

Stevens, K. R. (1995). Teaching vision and passion (Guest Editorial). *Journal of Nursing Education, 34*(3), 99.

Text of Cheney's *Report to the President, the Congress, and the American People* on the humanities in America. (1988). *Chronicle of Higher Education, 35*(4), A17–A23.

Vande Zande, G. A. (1995). The liberal arts and professional nursing:

Making the connections. *Journal of Nursing Education, 34*(2), 93–94.

Wilson, H. S. (1974). A case for humanities in professional nursing education. *Nursing Forum, 12*(4), 406–417.

Woditsch, G. A., Schlesinger, M. A., & Giardina, R. C. (1987). The skillful baccalaureate. Doing what liberal education does best. *Change, 19*(6), 48–57.

Zaborowska, R. (1995). Senior nursing students' self-reported college experiences and gains toward liberal education goals. *Journal of Nursing Education, 34*(5), 155–161.

2

Teaching Nursing Using Literature

Florence Nightingale's approach to the education of professional nurses included the study of scientific knowledge, training in the technical aspects of nursing, and attention to the development of personal values. In pursuit of the latter, the "Founder of Modern Nursing" recommended that her students read a variety of selections from among the humanities and encouraged them to compile a list of the literary works they had read. A review of the students' lists reveals that they read at least 10 books per year. Many of the works addressed the social concerns of the times as depicted by Charles Dickens and Mark Twain. Other books, such as assignments from the pens of William Shakespeare and St. Augustine, were intended to stimulate students' minds and foster character development (Schuyler, 1978). Because the objectives of nursing education continue to reside within the affective, as well as within the cognitive and psychomotor domains, the use of literature is as critical today as it was in the inception phase of the profession.

Literature, a discipline generally included within the humanities, is defined as "a body of writings in prose or verse" (Mish, 1990, p. 697). The physical and emotional experiences of human beings as they interact with people, places, and events in their daily lives are the primary focus of literary works. In addition to being a pleasurable experience, reading literature exposes students to the personal reflections of numerous authors. Through their written depictions of real or imagined phenomena, authors provide students with the opportunity to gain insight into human nature, to explore the realities of life vicariously, and to develop sensitivity to the needs and experiences of others.

Because human responses to health problems are the central concern of nursing, the use of literature as a teaching strategy to enhance the empathic awareness, that is so critical to professional practice, is most appropriate. Novels, short stories, children's books, and poetry are offered here as principal examples of literature. Comments regarding advantages, disadvantages, concerns, resources for identifying literary works, and selection criteria are addressed as they relate to the use of literature in general. Specific issues are included within the discussions of the individual forms of literature.

ADVANTAGES

The use of literature in the education of professional nurses offers a variety of distinct advantages. The most obvious advantage is simply the vast number of literary works that are available and the ready accessibility of many of these to faculty and students. Because the knowledge base of nursing derives from a broad spectrum of physical, social, and behavioral sciences, as well as from nursing itself, literature that addresses any number of developmental, interpersonal, and social concerns is worthy of consideration.

An additional advantage is that literature exposes students to quality writing and thus enables faculty to address concerns regarding students' abilities to write in a clear and concise manner. Also, the characteristic of creative expression is inherent in literary works. The relevance of creativity to the development of caring as a critical component of the art of nursing is described in the nursing literature and warrants serious consideration among educators (Lindberg, Hunter, & Kruszewski, 1994). Acknowledging that the experience of creative expression may be foreign to students, faculty can facilitate this ability by providing students with examples of creativity as it is expressed in literature. In addition, the solitary nature of reading serves to enhance introspection, an activity that is critical to the development of self-awareness, an essential characteristic of the caring practitioner.

The process through which information becomes integrated into knowledge is not understood completely; however, the appropriate and informed use of literature fosters students' appreciation of the value of non-nursing material to their personal and professional development. Although a number of authors support the notion of assisting students to integrate information, several caution that the most significant value is realized when the liberal arts are actually brought to bear within the major area of study (Boyer, 1987; Newell, 1989).

The use of literature as a creative teaching method "fits" with the current shift in nursing education from traditional, behavioral models of learning to an emphasis on faculty-student dialogue (Bevis, 1993). Active learning and more intensive class participation are outcomes of discussions based on assigned readings. In addition, students have the opportunity to improve their problem solving skills and to develop their ability to think critically and creatively as they reflect on the variety of interpretations and new meanings offered by faculty and fellow students.

Although changes in the content and process of nursing education are being discussed, many valuable aspects of behavioral models of learning will remain in the curricula. Literary works are adaptable as teaching strategies and evaluating methods for the various levels of behavioral objectives in each of the three domains of learning.

Final advantages to the use of literature in nursing education are that student interest is stimulated and the retention of content is increased when factual, technical nursing material is integrated with the human experiences described in literary works (Germain, 1986). Because the uniqueness of nursing lies in the ability of its practitioners to respond to the humanistic as well as the scientific aspects of health care, the opportunity to experience both in the classroom can only enhance students' capabilities as nurses.

DISADVANTAGES

The increased demand on faculty time may be viewed as a significant disadvantage to the use of literature as a strategy for teaching and evaluation in nursing education. Although it is not required that they be literary critics, faculty must read literary works critically for relevance to course objectives, accuracy of scientific content, and potential appeal before assigning them to students. An additional disadvantage is the need to advance-order sufficient copies of assigned readings and the added cost of book purchases to students.

RELATED CONCERNS

Several concerns need to be addressed when integrating literary works into nursing courses. Faculty must provide students with the rationale for the use of nontraditional assignments so that they will find meaning in them and thus achieve the intended learning objectives. It also is necessary for the teacher to prepare study guides in an effort to clarify the relevance of the reading and facilitate students' integration of the literary content with the nursing material presented in class. Additionally, evaluation methods should be developed that are consistent with the use of literature as a teaching strategy (Germain, 1986). Traditional multiple choice tests will not be adequate to assess students' achievement of learning objectives. More appropriate evaluation methods include such activities as written reactions to readings and student-led discussions of alternative solutions to problems addressed in the literature.

Another consideration is that specific class time must be allotted for discussion and debriefing periods. Without this important aspect, students and colleagues may come to perceive the use of literary works as "busy work," or as merely an unwarranted insertion of content into an already overwhelming curriculum. Finally, faculty should remember that literature should be used as an adjunct to, rather than a substitute for, basic nursing knowledge.

RESOURCES

Personal reading experiences are particularly valuable as resources for identifying appropriate literature. Familiarity with a specific work reduces preparation time and provides an opportunity for faculty to share interests with students that are outside the scope of nursing. One should also be alert to the potential for discovering relevant works when discussing reading with family, friends, and colleagues. It is a wonderful experience when a casual conversation yields an unanticipated "find."

Faculty from disciplines other than nursing, for example, colleagues in the English department, can be especially helpful in identifying works as well as in providing unique perspectives. Also, bookstore and library browsing provide a relaxing way to identify resources and offer the additional advantage of "combining business with pleasure."

Additional resources for identifying relevant literature include best-seller lists, book reviews, indexes, and anthologies. *The New York Times* publishes a weekly book review section in the Sunday edition that includes novels, collections of short stories and poetry, as well as the most recent publications for children. Also, faculty may find *The Reader's Encyclopedia* (Benet, 1987) particularly helpful. This classic guide to world literature provides information about novelists, poets, and playwrights, as well as synopses of major works and descriptions of central characters.

Many of the anthologies that are available provide brief annotations and categorize works according to subject matter; comments about several of these are included within the discussions of the specific literary types. Subject matter categorization is especially useful when seeking literature that addresses a specific concept.

SELECTION CRITERIA

Certain criteria specific to the selection of appropriate literature must be considered. Characteristics of literary works that warrant particular attention are length, accuracy and timeliness of the content, quality of writing as well as writing style, cost, availability of copies of the work, relevance to course content, and overall appeal to students. A work that cannot be completed in the allotted time, is of poor quality, or does not appeal to students' interests and learning needs will defeat the purpose of using nontraditional teaching strategies and only serve to frustrate students and faculty alike.

THE NOVEL

The subject matter of novels and the environments in which events occur are as variable as the experiences of life itself. Holman (1978) commented that the world of the novelist "may be only within the lowest recesses of the human unconscious [or]... it may be the fixed social structure of an aristocratic society " (p. 354). It is, in fact, the fictionalization and lengthy development of human experiences, and the variety of settings and topics unique to novels, that make them so attractive as creative teaching strategies in nursing education.

Although the length of novels is cited as an advantage in terms of the depth of character and theme development that they afford, length must also be discussed as a potential disadvantage. This concern can be addressed by carefully selecting specific, relevant portions of a book and by providing students with necessary plot and character detail. An alternative approach would involve assigning individual students to read and summarize chapters of a book; the entire book could then be discussed in a group session using cooperative teaching strategies. In an ideal situation, an interdisciplinary approach could satisfy the issue of length and address the learning objectives of more than one course. For example, students might read *The Great Santini* (Conroy, 1976) from the perspective of literary critique as an assignment in an American Literature course concurrent with nursing's use of the novel to examine the concepts of Family and Interpersonal Communication (Bruderle & Valiga, 1994).

Concerns regarding cost to students and the availability of sufficient copies can often be resolved through negotiation with campus bookstores or direct contact with publishers. Purchase price is often reduced when books are ordered in quantity; it is necessary, however, to allow time for delivery of bulk orders.

THE SHORT STORY

Holman (1978) distinguished short stories from novels in terms of the manner in which a character or an event is developed. He noted that in short stories, the true nature of the character or event is revealed through a series of actions; often, the actions occur when the character is in the midst of a stressful situation. Conversely, in novels characters develop as the result of certain actions or events; essentially, a process of development is revealed. This particular distinction suggests that short stories offer a unique advantage to faculty preparing nurses for professional practice. In acute care settings, in particular, nurses rarely have the opportunity to develop relationships with patients over a sustained period of time or to observe the process through which individuals and families respond to health problems. More often than not their interventions are based on rapid assessments with little time for deliberative decision making. The brief experiences described in short stories are not unlike the situations in which professional nurses practice today; thus they facilitate students' ability to identify with and understand human nature and to prepare themselves for the realities of nursing.

Although short stories were not distinguished as a specific literary genre until the 19th century, storytelling as a creative media dates to the beginning of time and reflects humankind's need to hear and tell tales (Holman, 1978). Again this unique characteristic may serve educators' goals. Most individuals have some experience with oral and/or written stories and relate well to this literary type as a means of describing and understanding human events and relationships.

The Short Story Index (Greenfieldt, 1991) is recommended as a guide to short stories that have appeared in collections and periodicals. This index, which categorizes information according to author, title, and subject matter, is published annually.

CHILDREN'S BOOKS

Currently there exists within children's literature a wide variety of reading options that render this category useful as a nontraditional teaching strategy. In fact, Younger (1990) suggests that simple stories provide valuable insights for a wide variety of age groups, albeit at "different levels of meaning" (p. 42). For example, children are drawn repeatedly to simple stories that portray human emotions while adults discover, in these same stories, relevant messages that foster their understanding of complex issues (Cardoza, 1992).

Although the simplicity inherent in children's books is more often than not an advantage in terms of representing human experiences, several considerations need to be addressed. Because such works are targeted specifically to young readers, the language and concepts will be limited to those that children are able to read and understand. It is important, then, that nursing faculty, when using children's books as teaching tools, acknowledge that the material is simplistic. Students also should be made aware of the value and purpose of such assignments. Finally, works should be screened carefully to eliminate those books that appear to patronize, condescend, or be overly sentimental.

There are numerous guides and booklists available to assist in the selection of children's books. Many of these categorize children's books according to literary type and/or historical period. *The Oxford Companion to Children's Literature* (Carpenter & Prichard, 1984) is a guide to children's literature from the earliest written legends to more contemporary works. This comprehensive reference includes authors, plot summaries, and characters from books, cartoons, comic strips, radio, and television. A reference source with particular relevance to nursing education is Bernstein's (1977) *Books to Help Children Cope with Separation and Loss*. The author includes annotations of 438 books that address such concepts as death, divorce, illness, war, homelessness, displacement, and adoption. Although written for and from the perspective of children, many of the books cited by Bernstein can provide students with vicarious experiences of situations that they are likely to encounter in professional practice.

An interesting and creative approach to identifying children's books is to ask students to describe their personal reading experiences. Imagine the pleasure students can have in sharing beloved stories from their childhood with classmates and in viewing these books from a more mature perspective.

POETRY

Poetry, an ancient form of human expression, is associated with imagination, intense emotion, passion, dignity, beauty, and meaning. Humans used the rhythmic quality of poetry to describe their responses to people, events, and the world around them even before the existence of written literature. Essentially, all poetry exhibits the qualities of content, form, and effect, and all poetry has pleasure as its ultimate purpose (Baldick, 1990; Holman, 1978), even though that "pleasure" may take the form of experiencing someone else's pain.

The literary characteristics of poetry such as arrangement, order, rhythm, pattern, and regularity are useful for educational purposes in that they appeal to the emotions and senses yet demonstrate a consistency reflective of the pattern and order of life itself. Poetry offers a "safe haven" for the expression and interpretation of those ideas and feelings that are often perceived but rarely expressed.

Poetry is useful in the classroom when introducing new subject matter. It can set the mood for a new topic, provide an alternative perspective on content, or offer an opportunity for personal reflection at the conclusion of a class session. An alternative approach is to use poetry writing by students as a means of monitoring their understanding of content presented in class. Use of this strategy fosters students' creativity and facilitates assessment of the entire group's learning (Peck, 1993).

In addition, faculty can use poetry to ascertain students' ideas and feeling by instructing them to write a poem or to select one that reflects their views. The availability of poetry, students' familiarity with it, the freedom that poetry affords, and its relative brevity combine to make poetry an attractive adjunct to teaching.

Initially, students and faculty may experience some difficulty with the use of poetry. The imaginative nature of poetry and the use of figures of speech require patience and the willingness to be open to new forms of expression. The advantage of such openness, however, is that future nurses may relate more easily to patients' emotional and personal descriptions of experiences such as pain or loss. Rarely do individuals describe such intense events in technical terms!

The Columbia Granger's Index to Poetry (Hazen, 1994) is a particularly helpful resource in that it facilitates the search in several ways. Poems are indexed by author, title, first line, last line, and subject matter. In addition, the guide lists over 400 anthologies and indicates which of these contains specific poems.

CONCLUSION

Faculty who are willing to expand their teaching repertoire beyond traditional methods by including the use of literature, foster students' ability to view information and achieve understanding from a variety of perspectives. When students and faculty discuss their literary experiences together, they create a learning environment that is distinguishable by a sense of shared awareness. It is this awareness that enables nurses to understand individuals whose experiences may be very different from their own, to integrate their experiences with those of their patients, and to provide care that meets individual patient and family needs.

REFERENCES

Baldick, C. (Ed.). (1990). *The concise Oxford dictionary of literary terms.* New York: Oxford University Press.

Benet, W. (Ed.). (1987). *Reader's encyclopedia* (3rd ed.). New York: Harper.

Bernstein, J. (Ed.). (1977). *Books to help children cope with separation and loss.* New York: Bowker.

Bevis. E. (1993). All in all, it was a pretty good funeral. *Journal of Nursing Education, 32,* 101–105.

Boyer, E. (1987). *College: The undergraduate experience in America.* New York: Harper & Row.

Bruderle, E., & Valiga, T. (1994). Integrating the arts and humanities into nursing education. In P. Chinn & J. Watson (Eds.), *Art & aesthetics in nursing* (pp. 117–144). New York: National League for Nursing.

Cardoza, N. (1992, March 22). Children's books (Review of *Journey*). *The New York Times,* 25.

Carpenter, H., & Prichard, M. (1984). *The Oxford companion to children's literature.* New York: Oxford University Press.

Conroy, P. (1976). *The great Santini.* Boston: Houghton Mifflin.

Germain, C. (1986). Using literature to teach nursing. *Journal of Nursing Education, 25*(2), 84–86.

Greenfieldt, J. (Ed.). (1991). *Short story index.* New York: H. W. Wilson.

Hazen, E. (Ed.). (1994). *The Columbia Granger's index to poetry* (10th ed.). New York: Columbia University Press.

Holman, C. H. (Ed.). (1978). *A handbook to literature.* (3rd ed.). Indianapolis: Odyssey Press.

Lindberg, J., Hunter, M., & Kruszewski, A. (1994). *Introduction to nursing* (2nd ed.). Philadelphia: Lippincott.

Mish, F. (Ed.). (1990). *Webster's ninth new collegiate dictionary* (9th ed.). Springfield, MA: Merriam–Webster.

Newell, L. (1989). The healing arts and the liberal arts in concert. In R. A. Armour & B. S. Fuhrmann (Eds.), *Integrating liberal learning and professional education* (pp. 67–76). San Francisco: Jossey–Bass.

Peck, S. (1993). Monitoring student learning with poetry writing. *Journal of Nursing Education, 32*(4), 190–191.

Schuyler, C. (1978). The Nightingale program for educating professional nurses and its initial interpretation in the United States. In M. L. Fitzpatrick (Ed.), *Historical studies in nursing* (pp. 31–54). New York: Teachers College Press.

Younger, J. (1990). Literary works as a mode of knowing. *Image: Journal of Nursing Scholarship, 22,* 39–43.

3

Teaching Nursing Using Television and Films

Television and films are enormously popular media that serve to transmit attitudes, values, and knowledge to society in ways that are unparalleled by other forms of mass communication. Through the stimuli of sight and sound, television and films are at once entertaining and enriching. They offer exposure to multiple experiences while requiring little intellectual or physical energy from viewers. Individuals can choose either to sit back, relax, and simply enjoy the programs and films, or they can become engaged in them intellectually, at various levels. No matter how one decides to partake of these electronic offerings, their impact is well documented as both powerful and persuasive (Chesebro, 1987; Coughlin, 1990; Madsen, 1973; Winship, 1988). The pervasive effects of both television and films on all aspects of human experience, and their ability to attract viewers of all ages, prompt their consideration as appropriate teaching strategies in nursing education. The following discussion addresses advantages, disadvantages, concerns, resources for identifying appropriate works, and selection criteria that apply to both media. Differences unique to each are presented separately.

ADVANTAGES

The public's familiarity with television and films as sources of education and entertainment is the most distinct advantage to their use as teaching strategies. Individuals are exposed to these media at an early age and thus are accustomed to and comfortable with the significant role they play in the modern experience. In addition, traditional-age college students are familiar with the use of audiovisuals in educational settings.

Through the sophistication of electronic technology, the dimensions of sight, sound, and color are combined into graphic depictions that allow viewers to experience an individual's entire lifetime, the ravages of war or natural catastrophes, or the evolution of a civilization, all within the confines of a 2-hour film or a 3-part television miniseries. The ability of faculty to include such presentations as assignments to facilitate learning is a distinct advantage when one reflects on the content-packed curricula of most nursing programs. It should be noted that such an assignment does not add to content but enhances it. In fact, when used as part of the repertoire of a creative teacher, the viewing of television and films can eliminate more pedantic approaches to presenting the same content.

That television and films are readily available to the vast majority of society is another advantage to their use. With the introduction and ever-advancing technology of videocassette recording, individuals can view films and television in the privacy and comfort of their homes, tape programs to be viewed at a later date, or replay and reflect on selected scenes as they choose. Thus, former disadvantages such as ticket price, length of programs, and timing that conflicts with personal schedules have all but been eliminated.

As do other art forms among the humanities, television and films offer an opportunity for a vicarious experience of difficult situations and legitimize the expression of powerful emotions. Through the talents and creative abilities of writers and actors, students are assisted to explore human life and their personal responses to it in a controlled and safe manner. Faculty facilitate this opportunity by providing carefully planned viewing guides and by evaluating student assignments in an open-minded manner.

In addition, the sharing of responses between students and faculty enables students to identify and clarify their own attitudes and values as well as appreciate the uniqueness of the experiences of others. Such an exchange of ideas and perceptions also fosters active participation and stimulates students' interest in the class. Having the opportunity to compare and contrast one's experiences with those of classmates enhances students' critical thinking skills. Also, this acknowledgement of individual differences is an integral component of the humanistic perspective that defines the uniqueness of nursing within the health care system.

DISADVANTAGES

Television and films are considered primarily as modes of entertainment; this perception can cause students, parents, and colleagues to question the academic value of class assignments that incorporate such viewing. A clear explanation of the purpose of the assignment, and perhaps an invitation to fellow faculty to participate, should help eliminate this concern.

Producers of television and films consider societal trends and interests when selecting subject matter for presentation. An additional concern, then, and one that should be addressed carefully by faculty, is the need of those involved in the entertainment industry to attract and maintain viewers. At times, the result of that need is the idealization of human concerns and the presentation of complex situations in a simplistic manner. Also, issues appear to be resolved easily within a prescribed time frame. Awareness of this concern as a possible disadvantage to the use of television and films should prompt faculty to provide students with an opportunity for critical reflection on and thoughtful consideration of alternative problem-solving strategies and less-than-ideal outcomes. In this way a potential disadvantage can be used to educational advantage.

The influence of television and films on society's values and mores cannot be ignored by faculty who must be alert to the potential impact of stereotyping related to racial and ethnic groups, sexual orientation, male-female differences, and developmental levels. Who among us has not been witness to the hapless bumbling of the contemporary parent, the random sexual behavior of the single female, or the mind-numbing inconsistencies of the elderly grandparent as all of these have, at times, been portrayed on television and in films? Again, faculty can use these portrayals to initiate class discussion and to sensitize students to the actual uniqueness within individuals and the differences among them. In addition, such discussions alert students to the harm inflicted on individuals and groups when nurses engage in stereotyping.

RELATED CONCERNS

Concerns related to the use of television and films as creative teaching strategies are not unlike those discussed with the use of other art forms. The rationale for the assignments should be clear to students, and they should be provided with study guides, or other materials, that assist them to link their viewing with learning objectives. Also, follow-up discussion of programs should occur as soon as possible after viewing and should be a structured part of the teaching plan. Attention to these techniques will help to reinforce the value of nontraditional assignments as adjuncts to teaching.

A final note regarding specific concerns is the reminder that students' responses to and perceptions of selections from among the arts and humanities are unique to them. In fact, this is one of the factors that makes such teaching strategies so useful in nursing education. There are no "right answers," and responses are as diverse as the human beings who experience them. Faculty who role-model this view teach nursing students as much about human responses, the primary focus of professional nursing, as any textbook ever could.

RESOURCES

Over the years the media of television and films have explored human experience in myriad ways. In fact, it is almost impossible to describe an aspect of life that has *not* been addressed from any number of perspectives. For example, relationships within families have been depicted from an intergenerational approach, from the perspective of cultural differences, and as role models for what "should be." Although there is a seemingly inexhaustible supply of television programs and films from which to choose, resources are available to help faculty identify useful works.

There are numerous anthologies available in the reference sections of university and community libraries to assist in the identification of appropriate films and television programs. Because many of these are specific to either television or film, they are included in the individual discussions that follow this general overview.

Reviews in newspapers, magazines, and on television programs like *Siskel and Ebert* also are helpful when seeking relevant offerings. It should be remembered that reviewers' opinions emerge from their personal preferences and agendas; thus, reading or listening to a review cannot be a substitute for actually previewing a work prior to including it as a class assignment.

Often universities and community groups offer film series that incorporate the showing of a selected work with a follow-up group discussion. Some of these series address a theme or area of interest for a semester or season; this is an added advantage when seeking works that relate to specific learning objectives. For example, a film series on family communication might include works that examine interpersonal relationships from various developmental and cultural perspectives. The added aspect of group discussion serves to enhance faculty insights and may even provide suggestions for classroom use. In addition to being particularly helpful to faculty who are interested in expanding their teaching strategies, film series are an inexpensive and entertaining way to spend an evening.

Also, faculty who teach Film and/or Communication Arts at local colleges generally are aware of upcoming film series and willing to share time schedules and locations of such offerings. In addition, they are invaluable resources for identifying appropriate films and television programs.

Students' suggestions are helpful, as well. They do spend time watching television and seeing films and are familiar with, at least, the more current offerings. As an innovative assignment, faculty might ask students to select a film or television show that demonstrates a specific concept and to provide a rationale for their selection.

Perhaps the most valuable resource for the identification of relevant films and television is one's personal viewing experience. The added advantage here is the familiarity with the work that allows faculty either to assign selected segments of a film or to show portions in class, and to provide students with sufficient background to eliminate their having to view the entire presentation. Of course, faculty should refrain from sharing their personal perceptions of the work before the students have the opportunity to view it and form their own opinions.

SELECTION CRITERIA

In order to use television and films as effective teaching strategies, faculty must select them carefully. This requires that potential assignments be reviewed in a critical manner. The time involved in this exercise helps to ensure that the programs are indeed applicable to students' learning needs, and not employed simply for the sake of trying a new approach. Careful attention to selection criteria also enhances faculty credibility among students and colleagues and offers the individual teacher a sense of personal satisfaction.

The content of a program should be assessed for its relevance to the learning objectives and developmental level of the students. Often faculty can tailor assignments to ensure consistency with course objectives by showing only the most pertinent segments to students. However, choosing appropriate segments and providing students with a context is time consuming, particularly when only a very small part is applicable. Faculty time may be served better by looking for a more appropriate alternative.

Although it is not necessary that faculty agree with the position taken in a film or television program, it is important that they are comfortable dealing with students' responses and conducting discussions that enhance learning. This is not to suggest that potentially inflammatory subjects should be avoided but that faculty acknowledge their own limitations and biases.

Technical accuracy and quality are important to consider when reviewing works as potential teaching strategies. Many television offerings and films present the psychosocial aspects of illness well; however, they sometimes fall far short in technical areas. The risk here is that students may remember only what they see, and may fail to evaluate programs in terms of what they read in textbooks or hear in class. A current example is the failure of programs to demonstrate adherence to universal precautions and the sometimes blatant disregard for patients' privacy.

TELEVISION

Noted science author Arthur Clarke asserts that "You cannot have a modern society without television. It's as simple as that" (as cited in Winship, 1988, p. 356). Indeed, it is difficult to imagine life without television, an invention less than 50 years old that nonetheless pervades every aspect of our existence. Even those who are not regular viewers are influenced by the presence of and discussions about this technological marvel.

The impact of television on an international level is apparent in that now more than 160 countries boast 750 million television sets. We are surrounded by visible television towers in cornfields and along highways and by invisible transmitters that float above us in space. In addition, it is believed that "for every child born in the world, a television set is manufactured" (Winship, 1988, p. vii).

When it first appeared in the middle years of this century, television evoked concerns that it would destroy the art of conversation and ruin everyone's eyesight (Weiner, 1992). On a more optimistic note there was hope that viewing television together would unite family members. Although the weakening of family structures and other social ills have coincided with the emergence of television, no direct cause and effect relationship has been documented (Winship, 1988). Despite early warnings about its detrimental effects, and current questions about its negative influence, television continues to be the favorite pastime of millions of people and to serve many useful purposes.

Advantages

The variety of programming types offered by television makes it an excellent medium for use as a teaching tool in nursing education. Also, the relative brevity of most programs facilitates their use within the classroom setting. An additional advantage specific to television is that with a bit of advance planning, faculty can tape programs that are scheduled at inconvenient times, view and critique them when time allows, and have a copy available for future use.

Examples of Use

Situation comedies and dramas address personal relationships, the communication process, lifestyle issues, and problem-solving approaches, to name just a few concepts relevant to professional nursing. Faculty using these in lieu of traditional case studies may find that students relate in a more enthusiastic manner to their "patients" and devise care plans that reflect more active involvement in assessing needs and evaluating outcomes.

An understanding of interpersonal communication, the strategies that enhance it and the barriers that inhibit it can be facilitated through students' viewing of a variety of the numerous talk shows that currently permeate television. Students can be directed to observe and critique communication factors such as verbal and nonverbal messages, the quality of questions posed, and the nature of the responses different kinds of questions elicit. They also can be instructed to comment on the presence or absence of effective communication strategies, and the effects of barriers to communication on the overall process. In addition, small groups of students can be assigned to watch different programs with the goal of comparing and contrasting communication styles when the entire class reconvenes.

Broadcast news presentations and the currently popular "magazine" format programs are useful vehicles to examine the many ways in which information can be communicated. The ability to provide clear and concise facts to patients and families is becoming increasingly more critical as the amount of time that nurses have to spend with patients rapidly diminishes. By observing "experts" in the field of information reporting, students can hone their own skills and develop useful strategies.

The simple messages presented in programs created specifically for children also can prove useful when introducing difficult topics such as loss and death. Careful screening of such programs to eliminate overly sentimental or simplistic offerings can yield some worthwhile material for educational purposes.

Finally, public television offers a vast array of high-quality presentations that should not be overlooked as potential assignments. Two representative presentations that are repeated on a regular basis are "The Miracle of Life" and "To Live Until You Die" (Matza, 1988).

Specific Resources

The two most accessible guides to television viewing are *TV Guide* and the Sunday-supplement booklets that appear as weekend inserts in all major newspapers. *TV Guide* is available at newsstands and supermarkets. Both publications provide local listings that include channel information and scheduling; often brief summaries are included as well (Weiner, 1992).

FILMS

Almost a century has passed since the first "moving pictures" appeared worldwide as peep shows and nickelodeons. When music and dialogue were first introduced in 1927 in *The Jazz Singer*, what began as a new invention evolved quickly into an international industry. Generally described as an art form and sometimes referred to as cinema, commercial films are an influential mainstay of popular culture that provide society with rich and diverse experiences (Leish, 1974; Madsen, 1973).

Advantages

In a manner quite similar to television, films offer entertainment as well as the opportunity to experience vicariously the full spectrum of human behavior. Few experiences have remained unexplored in films. Selections are available that depict birth, disability, interpersonal relationships, change, and loss, to name a small sample. This characteristic makes films particularly attractive to nursing faculty for use as teaching strategies. An additional and specific advantage to their use is that the length of most films allows for an in-depth analysis of many of the concerns that confront society.

Examples of Use

The impetus for using films as a teaching tool came early in the history of cinema when the inventor Thomas Edison wrote in 1910, "I believe that the motion picture is destined to revolutionize our educational system, and that in a few years it will supplant largely, if not entirely, the use of textbooks in our schools" (cited in Madsen, 1973, p. 441). Although Edison's words have not become reality, films do present faculty with a viable alternative to traditional approaches.

In addition to full-length films designed for adult viewing, the significant number of high quality children's films available also are appropriate as assignments. Many of these are animated classics that students may have viewed as children, and can now be appreciated and interpreted from a more mature perspective.

Resources

Annotated anthologies are readily available in libraries and book-stores and serve as helpful resources for identifying appropriate films. The publications edited by Magill (1980, 1994) are prime examples of such offerings. *Magill's Survey of Cinema* is a classic reference source presented in a series of three volumes that cover representative films released between 1927 and 1980. The format includes an in-depth analysis of each film and comments about elements such as production and direction, release date, and running time. In 1981, Magill began his *Cinema Annual* that provides reviews of films released in the previous year. The advantage of the annual publications is the addition of a subject index which facilitates the search for films that address specific areas of interest.

The Movie List Book: A Reference Guide to Film Themes, Settings, and Series (Armstrong & Armstrong, 1990) is a reference on films released during the era of sound. The book follows the format of an encyclopedia in that films are categorized under specific entries, including such concepts as occupations, themes, settings, and film series. Again, this type of categorizing expedites the process of finding suitable selections.

Finally, *Roger Ebert's Movie Home Companion* (Ebert, 1992) is included here because it is highly regarded as a video review book. Ebert, author of a nationally syndicated film review column, provides viewers with comprehensive critiques of over 1,000 movies, a guide to mail-order video dealers, and a list of publications related to films and home videos. The book is indexed according to film title, performers, and directors.

CONCLUSION

The social impact of television and films is widely discussed and researched by those who examine the factors that influence civilization. Developed originally as entertainment vehicles, both media have evolved into modes of mass communication and true art forms. Their appeal to viewers of all ages, and across cultures and ethnic groups worldwide, is without parallel.

The opportunity for students to experience the varieties of human existence through the dual stimuli of sight and sound, offered by television and films, is one distinct advantage of their use in nursing education. In addition, discussions generated from such viewing enable students and faculty to examine their own perspectives and to reflect on the relevance of ideas offered by others. Growth in terms of students' ability to think critically and make sound decisions results from such classroom interactions. The use of television and films in nursing education is, indeed, an innovative approach that requires sensitive awareness of applicability and the willingness to review potential works with a critical eye and an open mind. There is no doubt that this is an approach well worth considering for its benefits to nursing students and faculty alike.

REFERENCES

Armstrong, R., & Armstrong, M. (1990). *The movie list book: A reference guide to film themes, settings, and series.* Jefferson, NC: McFarland & Co.

Chesebro, D. (1987). Communication, values, and popular television series: A four year assessment. In H. Newcomb (Ed.), *Television, the critical view* (4th ed., pp. 13–50). New York: Oxford University Press.

Coughlin, E. (1990). Research suggesting how people experience television may fuel debate on role of mass media audience. *Chronicle of Higher Education, 26*(46), A5–A7.

Ebert, R. (1992) *Roger Ebert's movie home companion.* Kansas City, MO: Andrews and McMeel.

Leish, K. (1974). *A history of cinema.* New York: Newsweek Books.

Madsen, R. (1973). *The impact of film.* New York: Macmillan.

Magill, F. (Ed.). (1980). *Magill's survey of cinema.* Englewood Cliffs, NJ: Salem Press.

Magill, F. (Ed.). (1994). *Magill's cinema annual.* Englewood Cliffs, NJ: Salem Press.

Matza, M. (1988, June 9). Checking out PBS classics. *The New York Times,* pp. 11, 4D.

Weiner, E. (1992). *The TV Guide tv book.* New York: Harper Perennial.

Winship, M. (1988). *Television.* New York: Random House.

4

Teaching Nursing Using the Fine Arts

Nurse educators have many teaching strategies from which to choose to help students learn nursing and understand nursing phenomena. Among those strategies more commonly used are the lecture, simulations, case studies, role play, and gaming.

This chapter addresses the use of specific art forms, particularly what might be thought of as the more "abstract" art forms, to help students understand nursing. This discussion will focus on the use of sculpture, music, paintings, photography, opera, and drama as teaching strategies in nursing, summarize the advantages and disadvantages of using each of these art forms, suggest resources for locating works of art, and provide examples for the use of each in enhancing the learning of nursing concepts.

The discussion of the art forms is, in no way, intended to communicate expertise in the field. Likewise, the examples offered for the use of these art forms is not intended to be an exhaustive listing. Instead, this discussion introduces the reader to specific art forms and their strengths and limitations when used as teaching tools for nursing, and stimulates creative thinking about what nurse educators can do to help students learn in more diverse ways.

The use of more abstract art forms like paintings, sculpture, music, photography, opera, and drama has relevance to and a legitimate place in nursing education. Such art forms can stimulate the creative potential of students and faculty alike. In addition, they provide both students and faculty with an exposure to the liberal studies or humanities which serves to broaden their knowledge base. Using such strategies to teach nursing concepts can be an enjoyable learning experience for students, a challenging and fun teaching experience for faculty members, and a means to achieve greater student understanding of significant nursing concepts.

PHOTOGRAPHY

"Photography is now so much a part of our daily lives that our familiarity causes us to overlook it" (Freund, 1980, p. 4) as an educational tool. However, all three kinds of photographs—art, documentary, and personal—have potential use in nursing education.

A photograph is a representation of reality and, as such, the camera is thought to be "seemingly, both accurate and unbiased" (Freund, 1980, p. 4). It "'takes' what is put in front of it [and] captures the subject without further judgment" (Beloff, 1985, p. 23). But it is important to realize that the content of the photograph, the perspective taken, and the way it is developed to show different shadows or tones *does* reflect the biases of the photographer. Thus, "any photograph is only part of a truth" (Ashton, 1989, p. B60), and photography is not as "neutral" as once thought.

"In one sense a photograph promises reality and truth and scientific precision . . . in another it is the domain of art . . . [and] in yet another it holds magic and mystery" (Beloff, 1985, p. 2). In fact, Freund (1980, p. 5) noted that "the importance of photography does not rest primarily on its potential as an art form, but rather on its ability to shape our ideas, to influence our behavior, and to define society." Thus, it is a medium which offers many possibilities and can be used to convey a variety of messages.

The camera has enlarged our world in space and time and "helped man discover the world from different angles" (Freund, 1980, p. 217). It can enter the "secret" places of our civilization and our human existence, and it allows us to really look at what is around us and maybe "see" it for the first time. In fact, "photographs are . . . doors that enable us, if only briefly, to step out of our old ideas about ordinary realities and experience them in a fresher, more vivid way. . . . Documentary images [in particular] extend our sense of community with other places and persons and include them in our consciousness and our concerns" (Guimond, 1991, p. 12).

Over the years, photography has been used to document events and serve as a stimulus for change as a result of its "tremendous power of persuasion" (Freund, 1980, p. 216). Photographs have exposed injustices, such as child labor practices in the early part of the 20th century, poverty conditions, and the horrors of war. Few can forget the picture of the 9-year-old Vietnamese girl who had been burned in a napalm attack and was captured on film fleeing down a road with other children. The sight of the almost-naked Kim Phuc tearing off the remainder of her burning clothes certainly conveyed more information and feeling than any written report could ever have done.

Photography also has been used to shock people. For example, photos may depict nudes or vividly show individuals with diseases, such as AIDS or cancer, that society would prefer to ignore. This use of photographs stimulates us to reflect on our values, morals, and acceptance of others, which has been cited as one of the roles of the arts (Greene, 1995).

Photographs of individuals convey personal images, tell stories, and "enable us to trace the sameness of man" (Ashton, 1989, p,. B60). Additionally, they point out differences among people, circumstances, cultures, and experiences. Photography also has been used to suggest ideas without actually voicing them (as is being done with political cartoons) and it has been used to bring ordinary citizens closer to famous and important people. Indeed, as one author said, "we can all possess the icon" (Beloff, 1985, p. 10) through a photograph. A photograph can show us things we might never be able to see otherwise, such as the chambers of the heart or the impact of the famine in Ethiopia. Finally, a photo provides evidence of personal existence and worth.

Photographs are an important part of all aspects of our culture, and photography has become "the most common language of our civilization" (Freund, 1980, p. 218). When we look at photographs, "we bring to a picture a whole set of personal and social associations" (Beloff, 1985, p. 18) and we, thereby, give significant meaning to a photograph. Indeed, one author (Freund, 1980, p. 215) has said that the "most special characteristic [of a picture] is its immediate emotional effect." Thus, photos can be used in nursing education to help students reflect on their feelings, emotions, and reactions to people and situations, which is important if they are to provide truly supportive care to diverse patients.

Advantages

As a teaching strategy, photographs have the advantage of being readily accessible, since they penetrate every aspect of society. Personal photo albums, books and magazines about photography, photo journals, and general publications, such as *Time, Newsweek* and *Life,* all are sources of photographs. In addition, faculty members can produce their own photos of clinical situations, children representing different stages of development, or environmental conditions in an urban community, for example, without too much difficulty.

A picture is easy to understand and accessible to everyone. It is widely accepted and has an almost universal appeal. In addition, photographs allow us to "stop the action" on a situation so we may study it carefully, and negatives can often be enlarged, duplicated, or made into slides to increase their accessibility to a larger group. Photography is an art form that is familiar to everybody and easily transportable, and it can make paintings, sculpture, and situations available for study at the faculty or student's convenience.

Disadvantages

Photographs also have some disadvantages. For example, they may not capture the richness of a situation since they do "stop the action" and record only a piece of reality. Finding the right photograph can be time-consuming, and it can become quite costly to produce one's own photos and obtain albums, frames, or slide carousels needed to store them properly.

Summary

Despite their disadvantages, photographs provide many real advantages for the teaching of nursing. The recent Voyager project, for example, might stimulate an interesting exercise for nursing students. The Voyager interstellar project included the launching of a capsule containing 118 photos intended to portray a view of this world to any extraterrestrials that might find the capsule. Nursing students could be asked to describe or collect photographs about nurses and nursing that they would include in a capsule that might be found by people who know nothing about the field. Given the very personal meanings which individuals ascribe to photographs, the results of this exercise could be quite fascinating. Students' attitudes toward nursing, their understanding of the broad scope of nursing's influence, and the messages about nursing they would like to convey to others could be illustrated through such an exercise.

Photography is "inherently magical" (Ashton, 1989, p. B60) and allows for stories to be told. As a widely accepted, appealing, convenient art form, photography, then, has the potential for providing a fun and exciting approach to teaching and learning nursing.

MUSIC

"Today, more people listen to music than ever before in the history of the world" (Storr, 1992, p. xi). It is a medium with which most individuals are familiar and which has a great deal of appeal.

Although music is "the most abstract of all arts" (Wold & Cykler, 1967, p. 17), that abstractness may be the precise reason for its appeal. Unlike photographs, there is no reality with music. It merely provides a stimulus that allows each listener to interpret the words, the sounds, and the feelings conveyed in a most personal way, and thereby to give personal meaning to the music.

Music incessantly moves forward and carries the listener on by its flow. As such, it does not provide "a refuge of escape from the realities of existence, but a haven wherein one makes contact with the essence of human experience" (Copland, 1960, p. 51). Since nurses attempt to understand how individuals and families experience and cope with loss, illness, threatened self-esteem, and other health-related problems, a strategy that helps students "make contact with the essence of human experience" would seem particularly useful.

Aaron Copland (1960, p. 62) asserted that ". . . music that is really attended to rarely leaves the listener indifferent." In other words, music profoundly affects us. It heightens our sensitivities and stimulates us to think carefully about life situations, both of which are important to nurses.

"No culture so far discovered lacks music. Making music appears to be one of the foundational activities of mankind" (Storr, 1992, p. 1). It is tied inseparably to the social, cultural, economic, political, and religious patterns of a society, and it is an art that is "deeply rooted in human nature" (Storr, 1992, p. 49). As such, music is an excellent way to help listeners appreciate a culture's progress, significant concerns, and modes of expression.

Music also has other properties that make it a valuable learning tool. It has a "mnemonic power" (Storr, 1992, p. 21) that facilitates memory. It can bring about physical responses, create a sense of unity, heighten alertness, awareness, interest and excitement, and cause a general state of arousal. It also reminds us of the many forms of communication between individuals.

The music used in teaching nursing concepts can be classical or contemporary in nature, and students can listen to an entire work or one small piece of it. In addition, depending on the format in which the work is available (i.e., record, cassette, compact disc), students can listen to it inside or outside of class.

The melody in a piece of music conveys emotions and feelings ranging from anger and hostility to sadness and depression, or joy and happiness. Through the types of instruments selected, the predominantly high or low tones which comprise a work, the volume at which the piece is performed, and the intensity of the work, different feelings are conveyed in an abstract way. The lyrics reduce this abstractness, to some degree, by providing actual verbal messages; however, similar to the way in which the photographer's biases influence a picture, the particular words chosen for a song, the emphases given to certain words or phrases, and the emotions conveyed through the human voice (e.g., sniffles, a cracking voice, a growl) are integral to the message that is delivered and will influence what is heard.

The function of music, therefore, is not merely entertainment. "Music is designed, like the other arts, to absorb entirely our mental attention" (Copland, 1960, p. 64) and to encircle people by enveloping them and turning them from pure listeners to participants. Indeed, specific values are expressed and crystallized in music.

It has been said that the freely imaginative mind is at the core of all vital music listening. Unfortunately, in the process of learning numerous "technical" skills, nursing students may develop into concrete thinkers and lose their creative and imaginative skills. One objective of using music in the teaching-learning process, therefore, might be to allow the music to restore to the student's mind some of the emotional aspects of nursing's reality which may be clouded by the demands of technology.

Advantages

Music clearly has numerous advantages in nursing education. It is something that most people like, or at least can tolerate in one of its many forms. Most students in college, including adult learners, have been reared in a music-oriented society, with music playing at home and in dorms, cars, shopping malls, and dentists' offices, for example. Indeed, it is difficult to escape music today, since it has become such a natural part of most people's lives.

Music also has the advantage of being easily transportable, and technology makes it easy to tape-record almost any musical piece to play for a group of students. Although using records or compact discs may be more difficult, selections in these formats can be taped quite easily. Additionally, there is a vast store of musical selections from which to choose. Thus, nurse educators will have little difficulty in finding instrumental or vocal pieces to convey practically every conceivable concept.

Disadvantages

Despite these advantages to using music as an educational tool in nursing, there are some disadvantages. Perhaps one of the biggest disadvantages is an attitude—on the part of faculty members themselves, their colleagues, or students—that music is frivolous and a "waste" of class time. Such attitudes can begin to be changed by being certain the music selected is relevant, using this medium sparingly, and planning carefully (e.g., insure that all equipment is in working order, provide students with the words to a song).

Another potential problem in using music is that students may not appreciate the full significance of a given piece of music. For example, students who were born in the 1970s may not understand the societal conditions of the 1960s that prompted songs about the destruction of the world, racial violence, and loss of innocence. In such instances, faculty members need to provide the historical or societal backdrop for that piece so that students will realize its significance and it will enhance learning.

Finally, it often is necessary to listen to a piece of music several times before the ideas and emotions being conveyed can be appreciated. If music is to be played during class time and such time is limited, there may not be an opportunity for repeated playing of the piece and its full impact may be lost. This problem can be avoided by asking students to listen to the music before class so they come prepared to discuss its impact, or by selecting pieces with which students are likely to be quite familiar.

Summary

Music is an enjoyable and extremely effective medium for the expression of thoughts and emotions. By having students listen to others' music, they can appreciate various conditions of human existence. By creating their own music or lyrics, students can convey their personal ideas and feelings. In either case, there would seem to be a place for music in the education of nursing students.

OPERA AND DRAMA

Opera is unique in that it combines several art forms simultaneously: music, visuals, drama, comedy, ballet, painting, sculpture, theater, poetry, in addition to presenting history. Indeed, the interaction of words, music, visuals, and action can "create effects that are ravishingly beautiful, dramatically significant, and personally meaningful. No other art form does as much" (Digaetani, 1986, p. 4).

Unlike photographs which represent reality, opera is contrived and artificial, perhaps "the most artificial of the arts" (Digaetani, 1986, p. 2). Consider, for example, the individual who is stabbed but does not die until a lengthy farewell is sung; this is hardly an accurate representation of reality. But despite this artificiality, the feeling conveyed through that farewell does "reach the soul . . . [and] capture our imaginations" (Digaetani, 1986, p. 3), perhaps because words, actions and music together do what none can do alone. The poignancy in such scenes causes observers to reflect on their own values and personal reactions to the situation, both of which are relevant to effective nursing practice. Opera, therefore, has value in the education of nurses.

The synchronization of people's actions with spoken dialogue that conveys ideas and meanings is a characteristic of drama as well as opera. Instead of a character being described to the reader through the eyes of the novelist, the characters in a play come alive in very unique ways, depending on the actors' interpretations of the roles, and the observer is allowed to draw his or her own conclusions about the characters. In other words, "a play is what takes place. A novel is what one person tells us took place" (Barnet, Berman, & Burto, 1962, p. 10).

"Painting, sculpture, and the literature of the book are certainly solitary experiences; and it is likely that most people would agree that the audience seated shoulder to shoulder in a concert hall is not an essential element in musical enjoyment" (Barnet et al., 1962, p. 6). However, a play is what it is partly because of the crowd, or the audience. Because "drama is an art not only of expression but of successful communication" (Walley, 1950, p. 8), plays are designed to affect the audience. "By concentrating on effects, drama endeavors to enlist the active participation of an audience in meaningful human experience" (Walley, 1950, p. 10).

Advantages

The advantages to using opera and drama in nursing education are that situations come alive, and viewers can become a part of the "action" that unfolds before them. These art forms also often combine many forms of expression—verbal, musical, physical— thereby appealing to an individual's different senses or potentially appealing to each individual in some way. Finally, the use of these art forms in teaching nursing is a way to help students cultivate their artistic understanding and appreciation, thereby contributing to their broader, more general education.

Disadvantages

There are, however, several disadvantages to using opera or drama to help nursing students understand relevant nursing concepts. First, operas often are performed in a foreign language, are quite lengthy, and are not easy to understand; the operagoer, therefore, must "do some homework" before attending a performance to become acquainted with the work, be able to commit a significant amount of time to the experience, and be comfortable in the formal arena of the opera house. This is likely to make opera less than appealing to a student, particularly a very young student.

Location may be a limiting factor in the enjoyment of these art forms. For persons teaching or studying in New York City or Los Angeles, the opportunities to attend performances of operas, Greek tragedies, or contemporary plays are greater than for individuals in areas that are more rural or isolated. However, the theater or drama department in local colleges often offers performances of plays that could be used in nursing education, and they should not be ignored as potential resources.

The use of opera and drama also may be limited by the fact that many faculty members are not very well versed in these art forms. In addition, keeping abreast of what is being performed, selecting the appropriate work, and giving students the proper preparation before they attend the performance could be an extremely time-consuming and difficult task. The outcome of such an experience, however, could be quite rewarding, and nurse educators are encouraged not to dismiss the opportunities offered by these art forms.

Summary

Opera and drama are multisensory, action-oriented art forms that have potential use in nursing education. Faculty might consider having students attend a performance of one of these types of works, read portions of a play or dramatic work in class, or read an entire work on their own to identify and think about managing the paradoxes inherent in life situations.

For example, the difficulties faced by and the conflicting messages conveyed by the title characters in Wagner's *Tristan and Isolde* (1865), two young individuals torn between love and life, on the one hand, and the rejection of life and despair, on the other, might be used to explore developmental tasks, interpersonal relationships, or ways of dealing with intrapersonal conflict. Understanding the challenges of living in society with a disfigurement and the needs of the disabled could be greatly enhanced after students have seen a performance of *The Elephant Man* (1979), the true story of a man grossly disfigured from birth who grows up as a "side show freak" and then is befriended by a physician who shows him compassion and friendship.

By being exposed to opera and drama, nursing students could be helped to learn about and develop a deeper appreciation for various human conditions. In addition, they also would be helped to appreciate art and gain a broader perspective on life.

PAINTINGS

"A few drops of paint, deposited on a flat surface, can absorb the eye's sweetest moments" (Schier, 1988, p. 13). This statement captures the essence of paintings, for "if we have ideas to express, the proper medium is language; but if we have feelings to convey the visual arts may be more powerful" (Bruderle & Valiga, 1994, p. 133). Paintings are a most effective visual art form.

"All artists have the same intention, the desire to please; and art is most simply and most usually defined as an attempt to create pleasing forms" (Read, 1968, p. 18). Indeed, this representation of the visual world is the painter's expression of himself and his attempt to arrange shape, color, texture, and content in a way that will elicit a pleasing reaction.

When examining art, the viewer must have "a perfectly open mind" (Read, 1968, p. 35) because the experience of viewing and reacting to a painting takes place instantaneously. In fact, "art is not a code to be deciphered but an experience that awaits the sensitized eye" (Schier, 1988, p. 14); thus, an openness to the ideas and feelings conveyed through a painting is essential. Since viewers have the freedom to react to a painting in personal ways, this experience provides for a "liberation" of the viewer.

According to Read (1968, p. 266), "the function of art is not to transmit *feeling* so that others may experience the same *feeling* . . . The real function of art is to express *feeling* and transmit *understanding*" [Read's emphasis]. Since nurses need to understand their own motivations and the needs of their patients to deliver quality care, paintings could have a great deal of value in nursing education by stimulating such understanding.

Advantages

Paintings, as a strategy to teach nursing, have the advantage of allowing students to express their own interpretation of what a pleasing stimulus, namely, the work, means to them. A painting can be extremely detailed, allowing for a thorough analysis of the situation depicted; or it can be quite simple, allowing for a clear, unencumbered presentation of an idea, emotion, situation, or condition. There are numerous paintings available from which to select, including those on display in nearby art museums, housed in a university's art department, or on display in local libraries or other public buildings. There are paintings depicting nearly every human emotion and situation, thus making them relevant to many aspects of nursing education.

Disadvantages

There are, however, some disadvantages to using paintings as a teaching tool. Probably one of the biggest deterrents is their accessibility or transportability. The museum in which relevant paintings are displayed may be miles from the university campus, and the college's art department may have strict limitations on the opening of its collection to nonmajors. In addition, even when faculty members *do* find paintings that could be brought to the classroom, care must be taken in how they are transported and stored. This deterrent can be overcome, however, through the use of photographs or reasonably priced reproductions that are available in book stores, art galleries, and museums; such reproductions can be purchased and transported quite easily, and they also could be used to decorate the faculty member's office in between class uses of the work.

Summary

One would assume that the biggest use of paintings in nursing education would be as objects for viewing, studying, responding to, and analyzing. There also may be great value, however, in encouraging students who have the interest and talent to paint their own picture as a way to depict a relevant concept and express their understanding of that concept. For example, students may be given the option of writing a formal term paper, writing a short story, composing a song, or painting a picture to depict *their* personal perception of concepts like nursing's image, poverty, or loss, for example. Not only would such an exercise stimulate students' creativity, it also would give them some degree of control over the course requirements they complete, and it is much more exciting for the faculty member to evaluate the clarity of the meaning and understanding inherent in a variety of different forms of expression than to read a number of very similar, traditional term papers.

SCULPTURE

"Unlike paintings and drawings, which only suggest or evoke the third dimension on a two-dimensional surface, sculptures actually exist in three dimensions and have three dimensional form" (Rogers, 1969, p. 13). This is what distinguishes sculpture as an art form. In fact, the multidimensional characteristic of sculpture makes it an art form that most approximates reality because it has length, width, and depth.

While most other art forms involve the creation of a piece, sculpture can involve creating and building or cutting away. Indeed, Michelangelo saw two types of sculpture: "the sort that is executed by cutting away from the block [of stone, marble or wood . . . and] the sort that is executed by building up" (Read, 1968, pp. 245–245). Michelangelo believed the "cutting away" type of sculpture was the true one and the "building up" type the false one.

"Sculpture may be almost anything: a monument, a statue, an old coin, a bas-relief, a portrait bust, a lifelong struggle against heavy odds" (Hoffman, 1939, p. 19). It has existed in the form of buildings, "religious icons, tombstones, cult objects, magic charms, monuments, garden and civic statuary, portraits, and domestic ornaments" (Rogers, 1969, p. 2). Thus, this is an extremely versatile art form.

Wood, metal, stone, marble, ivory, and terracotta are the more common materials used to sculpt, and the material used reflects, to some extent, the culture and environment of the artist. As we explore museums, art galleries, temples, churches, and public places, such as parks, we can find examples of sculpture all over the world.

Advantages

The advantages to using sculpture in nursing education are that it *is* multidimensional, it conveys cultural insights as well as the specific subject of the piece, it is durable, and it can be touched and felt by the student. Even without actually putting one's hands on a piece of sculpture, one can appreciate different textures simply through observations.

Disadvantages

Sculpture's disadvantages are that, like several other art forms discussed here, it may not be easily accessible or transportable. In addition, faculty may not be aware of the works available that might have relevance for selected educational experiences, but such works are numerous as the following examples suggest.

SUMMARY

Michelangelo's "Moses," a 9-foot statue of a serious, contemplative Moses holding the Ten Commandments, depicts dignity and power; it could be used to stimulate a discussion of the concept of power. "Abraham Lincoln," the Washington, D.C., monument created by David Chester French, conveys thoughtfulness, leadership, and self-confidence balanced with doubt and concern. Faculty might relate this piece of art to its historical context and thus initiate a discussion of decision making, the congruence between values and actions, or leadership during times of great change and crisis. Finally, the sculptures, masks, icons, and other items created by the peoples of Africa, Native Americans, or Eastern European immigrants might be valuable in helping students understand different cultures and the values important in those cultures.

As is true with other art forms, sculpture can be used to express the appearance and/or reality of things, to embody ideals, to explore the unknown, or to attempt to create a new order of reality. It, therefore, has the potential for being useful in nursing education.

RESOURCES

There are many resources that can be used to find appropriate works of photography, music, drama, paintings, and sculpture. Resources for photography include *National Geographic, Life,* and *Aperture* magazines, all of which routinely display excellent photographs of various life conditions around the world. In addition, there are many photo essays—that will be referred to throughout this text, on topics ranging from hunger and famine to the family and AIDS. Finally, *A World History of Photography* (Rosenblum,

1989) provides a discussion of the uses of photography and offers many examples, which are categorized as portraits, landscapes, objects and events, or the social scene.

A faculty member can identify potential songs for use in nursing education simply by listening to the radio, tapes, or compact discs, by attending concerts and symphony performances, or by talking with friends. In addition, two books—*American Popular Songs from the Revolutionary War to the Present* (Ewen, 1966) and *The Rock Music Source Book* (Macken, Fornatale, & Ayres, 1980)—can serve as valuable resources. The first book provides the song title, author, and date; tells the history of the song, who sang it and the recording studio; and describes a bit of the song's content. The second book categorizes songs by "important themes of rock," such as brotherhood, changes, racism/prejudice, loneliness, self-identity, violence, and sexuality; it describes what is meant by each category and suggests related categories.

Summaries of well-known operas are available in *The Concise Oxford Dictionary of Opera* (Rosenthal & Warrack, 1986), *The Viking Opera Guide* (Holden, 1994), *The Metropolitan Opera: Stories of the Great Operas* (Freeman, 1984), and Digaetani's (1986) chapter on "The Standard Repertory: The Fifty Most-Often-Performed Operas." In addition, *The Concise Oxford Companion to American Theatre* (Bordman, 1990) and *The Oxford Companion to the Theatre* (Hartnoll, 1983) both offer summaries of many of the well-known, often-performed plays in American and world theater. All of these resources provide overviews of the works, their composers, the dates they were first performed, and major theaters where performances have been given.

Finally, depictions of numerous paintings and sculpture can be found in a wide variety of sources. There are hundreds of "coffee table" books available for many artists (Norman Rockwell, Mary Cassatt, Michelangelo, and so on). In addition, the four-volume *Great Drawings of All Time* (Moskowitz, 1962), the *Praeger Encyclopedia of Art* (1971), and the *Encyclopedia of the Arts* (1966) all provide excellent photographs of great works of art. Many of the paintings and pieces of sculpture are shown and depicted in full color, and often an entire page is devoted to each work. Thus, faculty should have no difficulty finding appropriate works of fine arts for use in the educational experience.

SELECTION CRITERIA

As is true when selecting literature, films, and television, choosing works of fine art to facilitate student learning must be done carefully. Without question, the work must be relevant to the topic at hand and not merely used to be different. In addition, it is important that the work of art being used is clearly visible to all students in the group at the appropriate time. For example, if a faculty member is pointing out some particular feature in a painting and only a few students can see that painting in a book that is being circulated in the class, those who cannot see the work will be frustrated and at a disadvantage. Thus, it may be helpful to make slides—particularly color slides—so that paintings or pieces of sculpture can be viewed by the entire class simultaneously. In addition, if one of the advantages of sculpture is that it is three-dimensional, photographs/slides of such pieces should show the sculpture from various angles.

When selecting music, faculty should be careful that the sound quality is good, that all students can hear it clearly, and that words are provided in advance or as students are listening. If a song has been selected for the message it conveys through its lyrics and those words are not clearly understood, students will be frustrated and will not benefit from the strategy of using music as part of nursing education as much as they could. Other criteria to use when selecting the fine arts—cost, accessibility, and congruence with the program's philosophy, for example—are similar to those already discussed.

CONCLUSION

The use of the fine arts, even the more abstract forms discussed here, has relevance to nursing. The overviews of the art forms themselves, including their advantages and disadvantages, should provide nurse educators with an adequate foundation for their application. This knowledge, combined with the examples given here and in subsequent chapters is a beginning step to using the fine arts to teach a fine art, namely, nursing.

It is hoped that this discussion will stimulate nurse educators to consider the use of opera, drama, sculpture, photography, paintings, and music in their teaching. It also is hoped that the use of these art forms will be an enjoyable experience for students and faculty alike.

REFERENCES

Ashton, D. (1989). The elemental fascination of portrait photography (End Paper). *The Chronicle of Higher Education, 35*(31), B60.

Barnet, S., Berman, M., & Burto, W. (1962). *Aspects of the drama: A handbook.* Boston: Little, Brown.

Beloff, H. (1985). *Camera culture.* New York: Basic Blackwell.

Bordman, G. (1990). *The concise Oxford companion to American theatre.* New York: Oxford University Press.

Bruderle, E. R., & Valiga, T. M. (1994). Integrating the arts and humanities into nursing education. In P. L. Chinn & J. Watson (Eds.), *Art & aesthetics in nursing* (pp. 117–144). New York: National League for Nursing.

Copland, A. (1960). *Copland on music.* Garden City, NY: Doubleday & Co.

Digaetani, J. L. (1986). *An invitation to the opera.* New York: Facts on File Publications.

Encyclopedia of the arts. (1966). New York: Meredith Press.

Ewen, D. (1966). *American popular songs from the Revolutionary War to the present.* New York: Random House.

Freeman, J. W. (1984). *The Metropolitan Opera: Stories of the great operas.* New York: W. W. Norton & Co.

Freund, G. (1980). *Photography & society.* Boston: David R. Godine, Publisher.

Greene, M. (1995). Art and imagination: Reclaiming the sense of possibility. *Phi Delta Kappan, 76*(5), 378–381.

Guimond, J. (1991). *American photography and the American dream.* Durham: University of North Carolina Press.

Hartnoll, P. (Ed.). (1983). *The Oxford companion to the theatre.* Oxford: Oxford University Press.

Hoffman, M. (1939). *Sculpture inside and out.* New York: Bonanza Books.

Holden, A. (1994). *The Viking opera guide.* New York: Viking Penguin Books.

Macken, B., Fornatale, P., & Ayres, B. (1980). *The rock music source book.* Garden City, NY: Anchor Books.

Moskowitz, I. (Ed.). (1962). *Great drawings of all time* (4 volumes). New York: Shorewood Publishers.

Praeger encyclopedia of art (5 volumes). (1971). New York: Praeger Publishers.

Read, H. (1968). *The meaning of art*. London: Faber & Faber Limited.

Rogers, L. R. (1969). *The appreciation of the arts/2: Sculpture*. London: Oxford University Press.

Rosenblum, N. (1989). *A world history of photography* (rev. ed.). New York: Abbeville Press.

Rosenthal, H. D., & Warrack, J. (Eds.). (1986). *The concise Oxford dictionary of opera* (2nd ed.). London: Oxford University Press.

Schier, F. (1988, February 14). Book review of *Painting as an art. The New York Times Book Review*, pp. 13–14.

Storr, A. (1992). *Music and the mind*. New York: The Free Press.

Walley, H. R. (1950). *The book of the play: An introduction to drama*. New York: Charles Scribner's Sons.

Wold, M., & Cykler, E. (1967). *An introduction to music and art in the western world*. Dubuque: Wm. C. Brown Co.

Part II

INTEGRATING SPECIFIC WORKS OF ART WHEN TEACHING SELECTED NURSING CONCEPTS

5

Aging and the Life Cycle

I'm glad I met her
She helped me realize this
That aging is life

— *Jessica Tinko*[1]

The life cycle is a continuous series of developmental stages that begins at birth and ends with death. The myriad changes that occur throughout affect all aspects of the individual and are mediated by hereditary influences, personal temperament, and ongoing interactions with the environment. Although the life cycle is an orderly and predictable process, individuals experience and adapt to the various developmental stages in their own, unique ways. It is believed that self-actualization is the primary goal of human development, and that individuals pursue their own maximal potential as they progress through the life cycle (Potter & Perry, 1993).

The aging process begins at the moment of birth. Viewed from this perspective, aging truly is a part of the life cycle. However, fears, myths, and stereotypes regarding aging have generated a great deal of misunderstanding about this inevitable experience, and it has come to be viewed more as a part of the dying process than as part of the cycle of life. The recent, dramatic increase in the aging population has alerted society to the need for an accurate understanding of the normal aging process and for strategies to assist in identifying and addressing the unique needs and strengths of the elderly.

Nurse educators who are preparing students for professional

1. Note. From Schuster, S. (1994). Haiku poetry and student nurses: An expression of feelings and perceptions. *Journal of Nursing Education, 33,* 95–96. Used by permission of Slack, Inc. All rights reserved.

practice in the 21st century have a responsibility to provide the theoretical rationale for nursing care of the aging. It is equally important, however, that faculty use teaching strategies that foster students' understanding of aging from a humanistic perspective and that stimulate their interest in this often neglected population. Irene Burnside (1988), an expert in the care of the aging, referred to this responsibility as "the need to combine what is known with what is felt" (p. ix). The focus of this discussion is the aging process as it occurs within the context of the life cycle. Examples from among the arts and humanities are suggested as strategies to assist faculty in achieving their teaching-learning goals related to the life cycle and aging.

DEVELOPMENTAL TASKS AND THE LIFE CYCLE

Essentially, developmental tasks are the challenges that individuals meet and the adjustments they make at each phase of the life cycle. The process of human growth, as achieved through various developmental tasks, has a decided influence on an individual's level of well-being. Successfully completed tasks provide satisfaction and enable individuals to move along the life continuum in a fairly consistent manner. On the other hand, failure to meet developmental tasks creates dissatisfaction that prevents individuals from moving forward. The way individuals proceed through the developmental tasks of life plays a role in determining the degree of satisfaction they experience upon reaching old age. The development tasks of aging relate primarily to adjusting to numerous physical and psychosocial changes, accepting loss as a part of change, maintaining a personally acceptable lifestyle that gives meaning to existence, and continuing involvement with friends and family (Eliopoulos, 1995).

DEFINITION OF AGING

The concept of aging is defined as a "complex biopsychosocial process" (Potter & Perry, 1993, p. 832). This basic definition combines the biological aspect of aging—that is, the inherent biological changes that occur over time—with the psychological aspect, that is, the behavioral adaptations that occur in response to environmental change. Additional terms related to aging include primary aging or senescence, and secondary aging. Primary aging refers to the normal biological process that has its roots in heredity, and secondary aging refers to the defects and disabilities brought about as a result of trauma and disease (Burnside, 1988). As noted earlier, aging, theoretically, begins at birth; however, in our society, the elderly are described, most often, as those who are 65 and over.

DEMOGRAPHICS OF AGING

Statistics regarding the dramatic increase in the aging population are staggering. It is significant to note that not only is this group increasing in terms of raw numbers, but it also is growing in relative proportion to the total population. Currently, one in eight Americans, or 65 million people, are over the age of 65. Within this population are 3.6 million people who are 85 or older, the old-old, a group that the United States Census Bureau predicts will increase to 12 million by the year 2040 (FitzGerald, 1995). These data demonstrate that not only are more people living until age 65, more are living well beyond 65, a phenomenon referred to as "the aging of the aged" (Burnside, 1988, p. 6).

Additional statistics indicate that there are 10 older women for every seven older men, and that because of differences in life expectancy and the fact that men tend to marry women younger than themselves, there are more widows than widowers. Although White elderly outnumber their peers in other racial groups, demographers suggest that immigration, improvement in life expectancy among non-Whites, and decreased birth rates among Whites will increase the proportion in other races (Eliopoulos, 1995).

THEORIES RELATED TO AGING

The complexity of aging and the unique ways in which it is experienced by individuals confound attempts by theorists to describe, explain, and predict the aging process. In addition, no single theoretical description of a phenomenon as complex as aging can address all of the influencing factors that occur within individuals or their surrounding environments. Theories are useful, however, as a means of organizing and understanding existing information and in providing questions for research. Current theories related to aging are characterized as either biological or psychosocial.

Biological Theories

The major biological theories of aging attempt to explain the anatomic and physiologic changes that occur during the aging process. They include the Free Radical Theory, the Cross-Link Theory, and the Immunological Theory.

Free Radical Theory

The Free Radical Theory is based on the existence of electrically charged molecules, known as free radicals, that alter the structure of cells and advance the aging process. Proponents of this theory believe that free radicals are produced by environmental pollutants and the oxidation of proteins, fats and carbohydrates. They propose that a reduction in free radical activity would slow the aging process.

Cross–Link Theory

Collagen, a protein-like substance, forms a flexible matrix within connective tissue that facilitates the smooth functioning of cells, organs, and tissues in the human body. The Cross–Link Theory suggests that as individuals age, these matrices become rigid and impede normal function. Research continues in an attempt to identify factors that cause cross-linkage, as well as strategies to reduce its harmful effects.

Immunological Theory

The Immunological Theory suggests that aging is caused by the failure of the immune system to regulate itself. As normal function of the system decreases with age, the elderly become prone to infection and cancer.

Because the aging process *is* inevitable, interventions based on theoretical perspectives cannot prevent aging from occurring. However, the biological theories do have implications for health teaching related to nutrition, exercise, and stress reduction that may prevent the occurrence of disease and disability among the aging (Burnside, 1988; Eliopoulos, 1995).

Psychosocial Theories

The psychosocial theories of aging focus on such factors as personality, lifestyle, and environment in an attempt to explain the thought processes and behaviors of aging individuals. They include Disengagement Theory, Activity Theory, and Continuity Theory.

Disengagement Theory

According to the Disengagement Theory, proposed by Cummings and Henry (1961), the elderly and society withdraw mutually from each other. This intrinsic and necessary disengagement benefits both, in that the aging individual has time for self-reflection, and the tasks of society are passed to the next generation in an orderly manner. Critics of this theory question whether or not the withdrawal is beneficial to the individual and society, and suggest that disengagement may, indeed, harm both.

Activity Theory

Havighurst's (1974) Activity Theory is a sharp contrast to the Disengagement Theory because it asserts that the key to successful aging lies in maintaining a high level of activity. The basic assumption of this perspective is that individuals' basic needs do not change as they move into old age. Although this theory is widely accepted, it does not acknowledge the numerous physical and psychological changes related to normal aging that may affect an individuals' ability to remain active.

Continuity Theory

Neugarten's (1964) Continuity Theory posits that activity and engagement in later life are determined individually and are based on lifelong patterns of behavior. Using this notion as a framework, a longitudinal study of personality and behavior patterns is under way. Preliminary findings of this study have supported the basic premise of this theory. The Continuity Theory is a more widely accepted perspective on aging, perhaps because it acknowledges the complex nature of the process and allows for differences among aging individuals.

Summary

The diversity among the theoretical perspectives on aging underscores its complexity and suggests that much remains to be learned. A general implication drawn from the various theories is that aging, just as all other developmental processes, has some predictable characteristics, as well as some that are unique to the individual. Systematic assessment and valid interpretation of individual responses are key to effective nursing interactions with the elderly.

NURSING AND THE AGING

Historically, nurses have had an interest in and a concern for the aging. Over the years, the profession has provided the majority of care services to this group, and nurses have been instrumental in assisting individuals to age in a healthy manner. That nurses are uniquely qualified to meet the significant challenges presented by this diverse population is evidenced by the growth of and significant developments within the clinical specialty known as Gerontologic Nursing (Eliopoulos, 1995).

A significant implication of the rapid growth of the aging population is that nurses will be spending increasingly more time with the elderly in a variety of health care settings. Although myths and stereotypes abound regarding the aging population, this is a highly diverse group. Only 5% of the elderly reside permanently in long-term-care facilities (Ebersole & Hess, 1990). Despite the proportionately higher incidence of chronic illness among the elderly, the remaining 95% of this population functions at various levels of wellness as active, productive members of society. The goal of nursing is to help elderly individuals identify and resolve their health care concerns so that the process of aging is a healthy experience.

The health care needs of the aging challenge nurses as they perform their multiple roles. As caregivers, nurses provide total care to the most seriously disabled among the elderly. However, whenever possible, nurses should encourage self-care as a means of maintaining the individual's sense of personal worth and integrity.

The aging population also has a need for nurses to exercise their role as health teachers. Although aging is not a disease, it is accompanied by changes in many body systems that require adaptation by the aging individual. For example, sensory deficits and changes in musculoskeletal function can predispose the elderly to injury. By teaching them techniques that enable them to adapt to such changes, nurses enhance their well-being and prevent further disability.

Counseling often is necessary not only for the elderly but for their families as well. Changes related to aging may necessitate the need for families to make difficult decisions for, but preferably *with*, the aging member. Nurses facilitate the decision-making process by listening, by offering useful information, and by coordinating patient and family collaboration with other resources within health care.

Sometimes elderly individuals require nurses to function as advocates. In performing this role nurses ensure that the individuals' rights are addressed, that they receive the care that is required to meet their needs, and that their dignity as individuals is maintained.

THE ARTS AND HUMANITIES IN RELATION TO AGING AND THE LIFE CYCLE

To provide competent and sensitive care to the aging population, nurses need an understanding of the entire life cycle and the aging process in particular. In addition, and perhaps more important, nurses need an awareness of the aging *experience* that cannot be obtained from even the finest authority on aging. The use of the arts and humanities is suggested as a creative approach to enhance nursing students' awareness of this highly individual experience. Because the following example combines a number of media from among the arts and humanities, it is discussed separately.

One general resource that incorporates a variety of art forms related to aging is *If I had My Life to Live Over, I Would Pick More Daisies* (Martz, 1992), an edited anthology of prose, poetry, and photographs. This collection includes a number of useful resources for teaching the life cycle and aging, particularly from the perspective of women's experiences with these complex phenomena, and it has wide use. The selections address developmental issues as they occur across the life cycle and focus on the private decisions that women make as they progress from one developmental level to another. In addition, the editor chose certain works for their relevance to the factors that affect personal choices such as, belief systems, ethnic and cultural identity, age, and gender. Perhaps the most significant reason for considering this book for nursing education is its potential to enhance students' self-awareness, a quality that is a prerequisite to the ability to reach out to others.

Literature

Novels

The novel *Dad* (Wharton, 1981) is a moving, in-depth description of aging and dying explored within the context of a father-son relationship. John Fremont, a busy executive, husband, and father returns to his parents' home to care for them in their last days, rediscovers his love for them, and gains insight into his own life and family relationships in the process. The book provides the opportunity for students to gain an understanding of intergenerational "connections," developmental tasks throughout the life cycle, the struggles that the elderly face, and how the aging process affects families who must care for elderly individuals.

Although *Dad* is 421 pages long, it is riveting and easy to read. In addition, faculty will find it useful when addressing a variety of topics related to aging including conflicts regarding nursing home placement, relationships among siblings and between generations, and interactions between families and the health care system.

Linda Manor, a nursing home in Massachusetts, is the setting for *Old Friends* (Kidder, 1993), a non fiction portrayal of the lives of the institutionalized elderly. The book focuses on the friendship that develops between Joe Torchio and Lou Freed, roommates at the home; it also includes "skilled and sensitive witnessing" (Harvey, 1993, p. H1) of the experiences of a number of the other residents. The author, Tracy Kidder, treats each character as an individual and highlights each one's courage and dignity.

Old Friends is touching, but because it is not sentimental, it is an excellent resource for use in nursing education. Faculty could use the book to introduce concepts such as loss, changes in body image, personal identity, and autonomy, and to initiate discussion about the ways these concepts are experienced by individuals at different stages in the life cycle. Students could be encouraged to share their own experiences with change, such as leaving home to enter college, and compare their experiences with those of the residents of Linda Manor. This exercise may foster students' awareness that although human experiences affect individuals differently, the understanding that fosters empathy with the experiences of others can be developed through reflection on and sharing of personal experiences.

Short Stories

May Sarton's (1995) *Endgame: A Journal of the Seventy–Ninth Year* is an honest and realistic account of the author's daily encounter with failing health and the disabilities of old age. Because the journal entries reflect Sarton's candid acknowledgment of her physical and emotional pain, they are not pleasant. However, the author's confrontation with reality brings her to an acceptance of "what is" and enables her to persevere in spite of her numerous infirmities. The book offers tremendous insight into the experience of aging from one individual's perspective, acknowledges some of the inevitable changes that accompany the aging process, and offers evidence of the importance of support from friends and family to the well-being of the elderly.

Faculty can use this book to initiate discussion of the aging process and to emphasize that individuals experience aging in very different ways. In addition, Sarton's descriptions of such physical discomforts as diverticulitis and lung congestion provide students with an understanding rarely obtained from a textbook account. Finally, the book may enhance students' awareness of the critical role that nurses can play in assisting the elderly to express their feelings about aging and to live full lives within the limits of their particular situations.

Missing Pieces (Benski, 1990) is a collection of short stories that captures the life experiences and memories of a group of elderly residents of a nursing home in Warsaw, Poland. Because many of the residents survived the Holocaust, their stories emphasize dramatically the impact of events on the experience of aging. For example, in the story *The Tzadzik's Grandson*, an elderly woman, upon seeing a newborn, muses about the grandchildren she might have had if her sons had survived the concentration camps.

The brief, yet poignant, stories recounted in *Missing Pieces* are useful to assist students in recognizing the need to "know" their elderly patients' "stories" and to identify the factors in individuals' lives that affect their attitudes and behaviors. Perhaps, through this book, students will ignore the stereotypes about aging that label the elderly as difficult and will, instead, recognize them as unique individuals with compelling life experiences.

The importance of understanding the elderly as who they are as opposed to what they have been is a critical element of *The View in Winter, Reflections on Old Age* (Blythe, 1979). In order to gain insight into the experience of aging, the author observed and essentially listened to a number of elderly British citizens. Thus, the "talkers" (p. 12) in this excellent study of aging are the elderly craftsmen, villagers, priests, scholars, and city dwellers that the author encountered while preparing the book. In the introduction, Blythe notes that the elderly become their own story tellers in an attempt "to piece together a true self" (p. 12), and that in their stories, they reveal as much about their current situation as they do about their past.

This book could be helpful as students prepare for their first clinical experience with the elderly. After reading and discussing some of the vignettes, students may be more inclined to *listen* as their elderly patients talk to them, and they may come to recognize the value of their patients' stories. During the postconference, students could be asked to describe their conversations with their patients, to comment on characteristics such as repetition, attention to detail, and comparisons between then and now, and to consider the relevance of their patients' words to their understanding of them as individuals with unique needs.

Children's Stories

The emotionally charged children's story, *Journey* (Mac Lachan, 1992), is an excellent resource for teaching concepts such as developmental tasks throughout the life cycle and intergenerational differences in dealing with loss. Journey is an 11-year-old boy who has been abandoned by his parents; he lives with his younger sister, named Cat, and his maternal grandparents. Narrated by the boy, the story describes how the family members attempt to cope with the loss: Cat gives away her possessions and becomes a vegetarian, Grandmother plays the flute, Grandfather takes pictures in an attempt to create a new family history, and Journey searches through old pictures in an attempt to find the past that he has lost. Ultimately, Journey learns from his grandfather that his parents are never coming back, that life can be fine without being perfect, and that love was there all along, he was just looking in the wrong place.

Another useful story is, in fact, a picture book designed for very young readers. However, Cardozo (1992) noted that, often, simple stories enable adults to deal with issues that may be too difficult to discuss in a more mature format. In *Just Like Max* (Ackerman, 1990), when Aaron's uncle becomes sick and can no longer work as a tailor, Aaron becomes his uncle's "hands," and together they accomplish many things. This story can help students to identify issues related to aging such as loss, change, dependence, and the need for social support.

Poetry

Although written for children, "The Little Boy and the Old Man" (Silverstein, 1981) is a poem that will, no doubt, evoke an emotional response from students. The poem describes a conversation between a child and an elderly man in which they discover that they have much in common. The boy laments that adults don't pay attention to him, and the old man expresses the same concern. After students describe their feelings about the poem, they can be guided by faculty to discuss the importance of the poem's message regarding attitudes and stereotypes about aging that can adversely affect the care that the elderly receive.

There are numerous poems that address a variety of ideas and feelings regarding aging. Because of the relative brevity of most of these poems, they are useful either in the classroom or in the clinical setting as introductions to new topics, as points of reflection within a lecture, or as concluding notes on which students can be requested to reflect in preparation for a future discussion.

"Generation Gap" (Jenkins, 1978, p. 56) is a poem that describes the experience of members of the "sandwich" generation as they struggle to care for their children, as well as for their parents. The narrator's daughter was cute when she fell down, but it was a different situation when his mother was unable to get up after a fall. And the poem "Medicine" (Walker, 1991, pp. 133–134) describes a young person's perceptions of how her grandmaother sleeps with her ill grandfather in order to be there to give him pain medication during the night. Each of the poems described above are useful to initiate discussion about caring for the elderly and to elicit students' attitudes about this aspect of nursing practice.

Several poems address the passage of time and, thus, are relevant to the concepts of aging and the life cycle. For example, a passage from Ecclesiastes, in *The Bible*, that notes that "there is an appointed time for everything," provides a spiritual and philosophical perspective from which to discuss the joys and sorrows of human existence. In addition, in "More About T. S. Wasteland," Munhall (as cited in Oiler, 1983, p. 86) shares her image of an elderly man whom she perceives as trying to keep time from changing his life. Although the poem addresses the ravages of time, it also expresses compassion and empathy.

Two poems that focus on the importance of nurses' sensitivity to the unique nature of each elderly person are "Sunshine Acres Living Center" (Krysl, 1988, p. 15) and "Look Closer—See Me" (Anonymous, 1990). In the first poem, a young nurse encounters an elderly nursing home resident in the hall. Because the nurse knows the man is Polish, she sings in his native tongue to him, and he begins to dance. The second poem, which was found among the personal effects of a deceased nursing home resident, is an old woman's plea to be recognized for the person that she is and not as a "crabbit old woman."

A final example of the use of poetry in nursing education is Schuster's (1994) description of students' haikus as a means to express their feelings about aging. The author designed the exercise as a creative teaching strategy to enhance students' clinical experience in gerontology. The students' satisfaction with the assignment was so positive that it was carried over into their maternity rotation.

FILM AND TELEVISION

An alienated daughter, a crotchety retired professor, and his wise and devoted wife are the central characters in the poignant and critically acclaimed film, *On Golden Pond* (1981). The strained relationship between Chelsea Thayer Wayne, played by Jane Fonda, and her aging father Norman Thayer, played by Henry Fonda, parallels closely the real-life experience of the actors; thus, the film is a candid portrayal of long-standing, intergenerational tension exacerbated by old age and the fear of impending death. The film is beautifully photographed, and the dialogue, although at times simplistic, conveys clearly the difficulties that families experience as they attempt to deal with crises.

Each character in the film could serve as an individual case study to foster students' understanding of developmental tasks across the life cycle. For example, Norman Thayer's anger at being 80 years old and his concerns about dying are barriers to his completion of the developmental tasks of aging. Students could identify those tasks that need to be resolved and suggest strategies to assist Norman to find meaning in his life.

The Trip to Bountiful (1985) is an emotional film about an elderly woman's determination to return to her childhood home in Bountiful, Texas, before her death. The aging widow, who lives in a tiny apartment with her disillusioned son and his nagging wife, "escapes" from her confining, unhappy situation in an attempt to make her way home. The actress, Geraldine Page, received an Academy Award for her heart-breaking portrayal of the desperate widow.

This film is an excellent resource for examining intergenerational relationships, developmental tasks across the life cycle, and the concepts of loss and change as they relate to aging. It also emphasizes the effects of childhood experiences and family relationships on individuals' lives. Students need to recognize the importance of such factors and consider them when assessing patients and planning appropriate interventions to address their needs.

The problems that adult children encounter as they struggle to resolve issues related to elder care are addressed in a sensitive manner in the film, *I Never Sang for My Father* (1970). Essentially, the plot focuses on an adult son who is about to be married for the second time, and his aging, sickly father who now requires care and attention. The son knows that he cannot bring his father into his new marriage but he is reluctant to place him in a nursing home. Although this film provides an in-depth analysis of a dilemma that more and more families are facing, it is extremely intense and highly emotional. Faculty considering using this film need to preview it, in a critical manner, to determine its applicability to their students' learning needs and developmental level. As the aging population increases at a dramatic rate, concerns about who will provide care for the elderly become paramount. More often than not, care is provided by elderly spouses, siblings, and significant others. At times, the individuals involved in such arrangements assume alternating roles as caregiver and care recipient, depending on the needs of their particular situation.

The Whales of August (1987) is a delicate portrayal of a situation that is not uncommon in contemporary society: one elderly individual providing care for another. In the film, two aging sisters, one blind and bordering on senility, live together in a cottage in Maine. Together they confront the difficult task of deciding what to do about their situation: giving up their home means surrendering their independence. Their dilemma is made more complex by their contrasting personalities: one sister accepts life with patience and hope, and the other is embittered by her situation and lives in the past. In addition to sensitizing students to the caregiving concerns of the elderly, this film addresses issues such as change, dependence, and decision making.

The very popular film, *Cocoon* (1986), is an excellent resource for nursing faculty. The film focuses on the escapades of three elderly residents of a nursing home in Florida. The three men, not content to play cards and grow old along with the rest of the residents, make every attempt to avoid the mundane routine of the nursing home. When they discover somewhat of a "fountain of youth" in a local swimming pool, they feel physically and emotionally rejuvenated, and life changes dramatically for them and everyone around them. Contact with space aliens provides the residents with the opportunity to achieve immortality; however, they will never be able to return home. Most of the elderly residents accept the offer, and at the conclusion of the film they are levitated into the spaceship to begin their never-ending journey.

Although this film is touted as a comedy and a fantasy, it does raise critical questions about the elderly, and about society's perceptions of aging. The film seems to indicate that aging is something to be avoided at all costs, that the majority of elderly individuals are unhappy with their lives, and that, if given the option, the elderly would abandon their families to pursue immortality. In fact, the one resident who chooses to remain behind rather than to spend eternity without his recently deceased wife, is viewed with sadness and pity by the others.

This film suggests numerous topics for discussion including

myths and stereotypes about aging, the influence of films on society's perceptions of aging, and the role that nurses can play in dispelling myths and assisting individuals to view the elderly as valuable members of society. Because the nursing home residents in the film depict a variety of personality types and approaches to aging, faculty could select any one of them as a suitable case study. In addition, students could be asked to match some of the characters in the film with elderly patients with whom they have had contact, and to indicate how viewing this film enhanced their understanding of their patients. Finally, students could be instructed to suggest an alternative ending to the film that would serve to portray aging in a more favorable light.

The medium of television offers a variety of perspectives regarding aging; some are quite positive and others are, indeed, very negative. The long-running situation comedy, *The Golden Girls* is an interesting case in that it is very popular among the elderly, and yet, the oldest character in the program is the target of much insulting "humor." Perhaps the program *is* so popular because it is easier to laugh about aging than to confront the reality of this critical stage of the life cycle.

In contrast to *The Golden Girls*, the equally popular *Bill Cosby Show* portrays a very positive attitude toward the elderly. The grandparents in this program live in their own home and function as independent and productive members of society. Their children and grandchildren enjoy their company, seek their advice, and appreciate the value of their wisdom and experience. Students could be asked to compare and contrast these programs, and to consider why such different approaches are nonetheless appealing to vast numbers of the viewing public. Again, the impact of programming on society's view of aging could be a most interesting discussion, or provide the basis for a reflective, written assignment.

Finally, faculty could request that students view a number of commercials on television, and comment on those that target the elderly as consumers. Students could be instructed to note the types of products that are intended for the elderly, and the advertising strategies that are used to attract and hold their attention. It also could be instructive to request that students note those products that are *not* "pitched" to the elderly, and to consider the role of stereotyping in advertisers' selections of appropriate products for the elderly.

FINE ARTS

Drama

The dramatic masterpiece, *Death of a Salesman* (Miller, 1949), depicts the tragedy of an individual who is unable to meet the developmental tasks of middle age. Emotionally devastated by the failure of his business and family life, the protagonist, Willy Loman, loses faith in himself as a valuable human being and suc-cumbs tc ultimate despair. This classic play is produced, on a reg-ular basis, by community and university theater groups; it is also available as a commercial film on videotape.

Because the play provides insight into Willy Loman's feelings, it can help to foster students' awareness of the innate desire of indi-viduals to self-actualize, as well as of the despair that some people experience when their life's goals are not realized. Students could be instructed to identify factors in the protagonist's life that pre-vented him from succeeding; an exercise that could help them understand the influence of family and the environment on growth and development.

Music

Ideas and feelings about the passage of time and the process of aging are described in the lyrics of numerous musical selections. Two songs, in particular, describe the memories of elderly individ-uals as they look back on their lives. In the song, "It Was a Very Good Year," for example, Frank Sinatra reflects on the various stages of a man's life in terms of the women he has known and loved. The concluding stanza reflects the man's celebration of a life well-lived.

Similarly, the song "Sunrise, Sunset," from the popular musical *Fiddler on the Roof,* depicts an older woman's musings about how quickly her life has passed from one day to another with both hap-piness and sadness. Reflecting on past experiences is an important part of the aging process. The thoughtful lyrics and comforting melodies of these songs can sensitize students to the need to encourage their elderly patients to talk about their lives and to lis-ten attentively as they share their personal experiences.

In contrast to the reflections of past experiences described in the two previous songs, "When I'm Sixty-Four," sung by the Beatles, describes a young man's projections for the future and whether his young lover will still need him when he's sixty-four even though she'll be older, too. The song, a positive look at the future, reminds listeners of the universality of human emotions; it may help young students recognize that their dreams and plans were once the dreams and plans of their elderly patients.

Expressions of regret about past experiences also appear in many songs. Often the lyrics describe lost relationships, or situations that "might have been," if different decisions had been made. The singer and composer, Barry Manilow, wrote the song, "This One's For You," in memory of his father. The song is a tribute to the love that he once shared with his father, and a lament for the things they should have said to one another. Harry Chapin's ballad, "Cat's in the Cradle," describes a father and son who were never able to find time for each other. When the son was a child, his father was busy with his work; now that the son is grown, the roles are reversed and he is too busy to spend time with his father. The father notes sadly, at the end of the song, that his son had grown up just like him.

In caring for the elderly, nurses do encounter strained relationships between adult children and their aging parents. The intergenerational tensions become even more apparent when end-of-life and/or life-care decisions need to be made. Although nurses are not expected to reunite families, it is important that they have a sensitivity to the underlying feelings that affect attitudes, behaviors, and decisions. Discussion about the emotions described in these songs may expand students' awareness of the life experiences that aging individuals and their families bring to bear on their current situations.

Painting

The classic painting, "Portrait of the Artist's Mother" by James McNeill Whistler, could serve as a focal point for a discussion of students' attitudes toward the elderly. In this scene from the 19th century, an old woman, drawn in profile, appears serene and comfortable; her hands are folded on her lap, and her feet are elevated on a low stool. Although this portrayal of an elderly person appears to be outdated, it is not unlikely that some students continue to view aging in much the same manner in which it was depicted by Whistler. As students share their ideas, faculty should remember that the goal of the discussion is not to change students' perceptions, but to help them recognize that stereotyping is a barrier to understanding the differences among individuals.

"The Old Man and His Grandson," by Domenico Ghirlandaio, is both a realistic depiction of the physical differences between the generations and a beautiful statement of the love and understanding that can link the young with the old. In the painting, a young, soft-skinned child gazes fondly into the age-worn, scarred face of his grandfather. The child's hand rests on his grandfather's chest in a pose that suggests acceptance and trust. This painting might be useful to allay students' fears prior to their first clinical encounter with the elderly. In addition, it may help them to recognize the "gifts" that one generation can share with another.

Photography

The Family of Man (Saudberg, 1955) is an anthology of black and white photographs that depict individuals at various stages of the life cycle. Despite the age of this publication, the photographs are timeless and poignant, and the book is worth considering for use in nursing education. *A Day in the Life of America* (Smolan & Cohen, 1986) is a collection of photographs taken in the United States on May 2, 1986. Several photographs are particularly useful to faculty teaching aging. Because the pictures are untitled, they are designated for reference by page number: two elderly women resting on a bench in Central Park (p.78), 63-year-old bachelor twins having coffee in Oxford, Mississippi (p.79), and 85-year-old B.T. Wrinkle and his bedridden wife (p.150). Each of these color photographs depict elderly individuals in their own environments; thus, the pictures serve as reminders that the elderly have homes, families, and concerns that need to be acknowledged as part of their total being and plan of care.

CONCLUSION

Individuals experience the changes that occur within the life cycle in unique and different ways. Factors such as temperament, heredity, and environment influence a person's ability to move smoothly from one developmental stage to the next. The complex and inevitable process of aging is a critical aspect of the life cycle; often, however, it is viewed with fear and misunderstanding.

Nursing students need information about human development, the life cycle, and aging, but they also need an understanding of the meaning of life's experiences so they can provide care that is not only theoretically sound but also humanistic. The use of selections from among the arts and humanities is suggested as an approach to enhance students' ability to understand and care for individuals at all stages of the life cycle, and to stimulate their interest in the care of the elderly, in particular.

REFERENCES

Ackerman, K. (1990). *Just like Max*. New York: Knopf.

Anonymous. (1990, July). Look closer-See me. *Nursing Homes*, 34.

Benski, S. (1990). *Missing pieces*. New York: Harcourt Brace Jovanovich.

Blythe, R. (1979). *The view in winter*. New York: Harcourt Brace Jovanovich.

Burnside, I. (Ed.). (1988). *Nursing and the aged: A self-care approach*. New York: McGraw-Hill.

Cardozo, N. B. (1992, March 22). Children's books (Review of *Journey*). *The New York Times*, p. 25.

Cummings, E., & Henry, W. (1961). *Growing old: The process of disengagement*. New York: Basic Books.

Ebersole, P., & Hess, P. (1990). *Toward healthy aging: Human needs and nursing response* (3rd ed.). St. Louis, MO: Mosby.

Eliopoulos, C. (1995). *Manual of gerontologic nursing*. St. Louis, MO: Mosby.

FitzGerald, F. (1995, March 2). Test predicts how older people will age. *The Philadelphia Inquirer*, p. A2.

Harvey, B. (1993, September 19). Touching portraits from the full-of-life Linda Manor. *The Philadelphia Inquirer*, pp. H1, H4.

Havighurst, R. (1974). *Developmental tasks and education*. New York: McKay.

Jenkins, B.L. (1978). Generation gap. *Journal of Gerontological Nursing, 4*, 56.

Kidder, T. (1993). *Old friends*. Boston: Houghton Mifflin.

Krysl, M. (1988). Existential moments of caring: Facets of nursing and social support. *Advances in Nursing Science, 10*(2), 12–17.

Mac Lachlan, P. (1992). *Journey*. New York: Delacorte.

Martz, S. (Ed.). (1992). *If I had my life to live over, I would pick more daisies*. Watsonville, CA: Papier–Mache Press.

Miller, A. (1949). *Death of a salesman.* New York: Viking Press.

Neugarten, B. (1964). *Personality in middle and late life.* New York: Atherton.

Oiler, C. (1983). Nursing reality as reflected in nurses' poetry. *Perspectives in psychiatric care, 21*(3), 81–89.

Potter, P., & Perry, A. (1993). *Fundamentals of nursing* (3rd ed.). St. Louis, MO: Mosby.

Sarton, M. (1995). *Endgame: A journal of the seventy-ninth year.* New York: W.W. Norton.

Saudberg, C. (1955). *The family of man.* New York: The Museum of Modern Art.

Schuster, S. (1994). Haiku poetry and student nurses: An expression of feelings and perceptions. *Journal of Nursing Education, 33,* 95–96.

Silverstein, S. (1981). The little boy and the old man. In S. Silverstein, *A light in the attic* (p. 95). New York: Harper & Row.

Smolan, R., & Cohen, D. (Eds.). (1986). *A day in the life of America.* New York: Collins.

Walker, A. (1991). Medicine. In A. Walker, *Her blue body everything we know: Earthling poems , 1965–1990* (pp. 133–134). San Diego: Harcourt Brace Jovanovich.

Wharton, W. (1981). *Dad.* New York: Avon.

6

Assessment

Marycarol McGovern, PhD, RN

Most nurses would describe the essence of nursing practice as the promotion of health and the prevention of illness. The professional behavior of nurses is directed toward health and the health-seeking activities of individuals, families, and communities. Since the goal of nursing is the promotion of health, it is important to understand how nurses determine a person's level of health or illness, degree of risk, and need for professional intervention. What does the nurse know about this patient? What are the patient's needs? What does the nurse want to do with and for the patient? What does she want the patient to do for himself? Nurses come to these decisions by a process of assessment.

Assessment is the key that unlocks the essence and challenge of professional nursing practice. Nurses assess more than just physical status; indeed, since the nature of nursing practice is to consider the holistic nature of the individual, both actual and potential health problems, as well as the abilities to cope with and manage them, need to be addressed. But what is the nature of the assessment process? What do students really need to understand about the content and process of assessment? How can it be characterized, described, and captured to convey it to students who must master the art of assessment if they are to master the science of nursing?

Most nursing texts do not define assessment per se, other than to characterize it as the first step of the nursing process. Authors talk about assessment as it relates to other topics under discussion, such as cardiac, family, or mental health assessment; and Tables of Contents in textbooks advise the reader to *See Specific Subject* or *See Physical Examination* or *See Nursing Process*. But assessment is more than physical examination and more than a functional appraisal. Assessment needs to be considered from a phenomenological perspective, that is, from the context of the person's lived experience and future goals. Certainly the concept of assessment cannot exist in a vacuum; we assess something. But there is merit in reflecting on what the concept of assessment encompasses: what it is, what professional nursing knowledge and activities are involved, and how it fits into the total picture of nursing care delivery.

Assessment has been described as the collection, validation, organization, and documentation of information related to the patient's health status (Kozier, Erb, Blais, & Wilkinson, 1995). There is nothing inaccurate about this definition, but one must question if it captures the essence of assessment? Does this definition clarify the breadth and depth of the concept in its most humanistic sense? Does it lead to an understanding of the person's feelings and values as well as his physical responses? The nurse's view of the goals and processes of assessment affect how and what is assessed, how questions to determine the person's health status are asked, and whether the questions are asked to discover the individual's perception of his condition or illness. Perhaps a definition that addresses more than the activities of assessment, a definition that focuses on the context and concept of not just *doing* assessment, but *thinking* assessment, is needed.

ASSESSMENT DEFINED

Assessment is a caring, informed, contextual, reflective, and purposeful investigation of a patient situation; it encompasses the factors which affect the person's health and function, and includes the person's perception of his strengths, risk factors, and problems related to health and optimal functioning.

Assessment is Caring

Assessment needs to be caring. Nursing has been described as the science of caring; "to call nursing the health science of caring is to value health and its promotion, to emphasize the science of nursing as well as the art, and to acknowledge that caring is a prime interpersonal interaction" (Lindberg, Hunter, & Kruszewski, 1994,

p. 50). Caring is a prerequisite for comprehensive nursing practice; it implies that the nurse recognizes the intrinsic worth of individuals and their potential for self-care and for growth. It is especially important to connect caring to the concept of assessment to place emphasis on the person being assessed more than on the data base being developed. The nurse who *cares* for the patient is committed to excellent practice, and will engage in behaviors that insure that the information gathered and the care provided will be competent, thorough, and focused on well-defined patient needs. Caring involves attentive, skillful behaviors that focus on the patient's needs, decrease patient anxiety, and provide for a reciprocal interchange among patient, family, and nurse (Burfitt, Greiner, & Miers, 1993).

In order for nurses to develop an accurate, complete, and patient-centered data base, a caring approach is necessary to establish an atmosphere of trust and openness. Whether assessing an individual, a family, or a community, gaining entrance and acceptance into that patient system presents an initial and important challenge. If nurses are viewed only as agents of the health care system, their motives may be questioned, and the information which results from the assessment may be incomplete or even erroneous. But if nurses can convey a sincere interest in the patient and in the impact of health and illness on his or her life, they can collect and interpret assessment data which will lead to an effective, patient-centered plan that, in turn, will improve the patient's health and well-being.

Nurses establish an atmosphere of trust by demonstrating acceptance of and genuine interest in the person, by respecting the person's need for privacy, by incorporating the person's statements and feelings into the process, by letting the person know that he or she will retain control over the decisions that are made, and by helping the person identify and access appropriate support and resources.

Assessment is Informed

Assessment should be informed. The nurse must approach the assessment process in a knowledgeable, systematic, and comprehensive manner. Safe and efficient assessment involves the skillful application of the processes of inspection, palpation, percussion, and auscultation, as well as an understanding of wellness and human disease processes in the context of individual, family, and community health and illness. Most health care agencies, whether hospital- or community-based, employ a nursing assessment tool or guide which focuses on the unique health care needs of that patient population. Standard I of the American Nurses Association's *Standards of Clinical Nursing Practice* (1991) outlines the nurse's accountability for collecting, prioritizing, and documenting patient health data. In a legal context, assessment errors, including the failure to recognize significant and relevant data, are a major cause of negligence (Calfee, 1991). Thus, the nurse must be informed about the content of the nursing assessment and the process of professional nursing assessment.

An understanding of the skills of physical examination is important. It also is important to examine the data base for inconsistencies and for missing information. Reasoning skills are used to determine the relevance and validity of information, to recognize patterns and relationships among the data and categorize them, to develop areas for further investigation, and to refer the patient to appropriate resources for continued examination, care, and follow-up. All nursing activities depend on an accurate and complete assessment, since an incomplete or inaccurate assessment affects all other aspects of the plan of care. Establishing goals, planning and implementing nursing activities, and evaluating patient responses to health care interventions and changes in health status will be an incomplete or inaccurate endeavor if the assessment is not competent and comprehensive.

Assessment is Contextual

Assessment should be contextual. A context-driven approach is necessary since people interpret their experiences from their own frame of reference or view of reality. Since assessment is perceived as a holistic, patient-centered activity, the developmental and sociocultural characteristics of the person or group must be considered, as well as the relevance of data to prior realities of health, family, and function. When nurse educators ask students to consider the context of a patient's life, it is helpful to ask them to imagine various scenarios that may have taken place or that could occur, and to be open to the discovery of family and cultural dynamics.

Perceptions of health and illness, and the way in which people make decisions about their health, involve purposive behaviors that give meaning to experience. Individuals at different stages of development and with different life experiences think about health, values, and responsibility in different ways, and those differences are reflected in their lifestyle, their approach to health and personal fulfillment, and their decision making. Since individuals create their own reality, it is important for the nurse to assess what that reality entails and what goals are important to the individual.

When an informant other than the patient is utilized as a data source, valuable information about the person's health and physical status can be gathered, but it also is helpful to consider other data or pictures that emerge. Parents, of course, must provide data on infants and young children; other caregivers may be informants for children and ill or elderly persons. With both parent (or caregiver) and child present, it is possible to obtain the health history and physical examination and to observe the quality of the parent-child (or caregiver-patient) interaction. It is important to realize that parents and caregivers have their own assumptions, perceptions, biases, and needs (Bates, Bickley, & Hoekelman, 1995). Nurses must evaluate the frame of reference of informants, and consider the context of their relationship with the patient and with the problem being investigated. Efforts to establish a supportive, nonjudgmental atmosphere when interacting with informants as well as with patients themselves are important to facilitate communication and to discover meaningful information. The nurse who focuses on the holistic nature of persons and families will recognize that seemingly "peripheral" information obtained during an open discussion may reveal relevant data that are important in the decision-making process and may, in fact, lead parents and caregivers to express other, or perhaps even the "real," reasons for their contact with a health care professional.

In terms of context, it is necessary to ask, "Is this a normal or expected pattern response for this person as it relates to his age, culture, health problem, or lifestyle?" or, "Is this a change from previously collected data?" (Alfaro-LeFevre, 1995). For example, a pulse rate of 54 is not typically considered "normal," and the nurse must investigate whether the person is taking any cardiac medications, has had recent periods of dizziness, or engages in frequent aerobic exercise. If the person has foot ulcers which will not heal, the nurse would need to determine whether or not he or she has a history of diabetes or peripheral vascular disease; however, it is just as important to determine the hygiene practices of the person, family, or cultural reference group, the occupational and other responsibilities of the person, or even the type of footwear worn. "Providing culturally congruent care should be one of the highest priorities of nursing organizations and educational institutions as they plan for health care reform and to function in a multicultural world. . . . Nurses will be required to provide truly holistic care informed by knowledge of different world views and environmental conditions" (Leininger, 1994, p. 255).

Assessment is Reflective

Assessment should be reflective. Since health status is both dynamic and adaptive, nurses should bring a spirit of inquiry to the assessment process. There should be a curiosity about what is, what might be, what could be, and what ought to be, in terms of personal health, family function, and community resources. A tool for health assessment must be comprehensive, but it also should be flexible. It should allow nurses to utilize their unique talents and skills, and it should not limit their thoughtful evaluation of the data and the person's perception of his health status. Since each individual's experience is unique and complex, a single solution or approach cannot be formulated for every problem. It is important to remain open to alternate types and sources of data, and to interpret this information through a reasoning process that reflects each person's unique situation (Jones & Brown, 1993; Stanhope & Lancaster, 1988).

Because nursing defines itself as the practice of health care that focuses on human responses to health and illness, a linear approach to assessing and solving a person's health-related needs is ineffective. An interactive, dynamic approach is necessary to determine what alternatives and choices are suitable from the patient's frame of reference, and to preserve both patient and nurse autonomy. The person's own lived experience demands that the assumptions of both the person and the nurse are accounted for, that alternative solutions are not only tolerated but generated, that a clear rationale for action and decision is offered, and that conclusions are open to reinterpretation and negotiation. This process of "figuring out what to believe or do about a situation, phenomenon, or problem for which no single definitive answer exists" has been termed critical thinking (Kurfiss, 1988, p. 42). Critical thinking involves the way in which people make meaning, interpret their world, identify underlying assumptions, articulate a point of view, justify their beliefs and actions, make decisions and commitments, and consider the consequences of their decisions. In this context of critical thinking, it is important that nurses consider their own values and biases and actively examine underlying assumptions about patients and their situations. Relating the concepts of critical thinking and assessment implies a multidimensional cognitive process, rather than a unidimensional, linear process based on the "rules" of logic or even of the nursing process (Jones & Brown, 1993).

A reflective or critical thinking approach is not an "add-on" or a buzzword approach; instead, it is the method of reasoning and problem solving that is humane and the essence of nursing practice. Critical thinking is a good description for the process of reasoning that is necessary in professional nursing assessment. Critical thinking has been defined as purposeful and goal directed (Halpern, 1984), reasonable and reflective (Ennis, 1987), and a process that integrates all available information (Kurfiss, 1988). In fact, the relationship between knowledge and action is mediated by critical reflection (Ford & Profetto–McGrath, 1994). Once people are open to uncertainty and diverse perspectives, they can make sense or meaning out of an intellectual or ethical dilemma by using this reflective reasoning process that has come to be known as critical thinking. Thus, it is an invaluable skill in the assessment process.

Assessment is Purposive

Benner (1984) noted that professional nursing judgment is an acquired skill that depends on past experience. Expert competence, the highest level of proficiency, is characterized by assessing alternatives and considering multiple alternatives and by conscious, deliberate planning. This purposive dimension is important to an understanding of the process and outcomes of assessment. Nurse educators can present the problem-solving aspect of assessment as a goal, thereby helping students understand that assessment is not just a compilation of facts and even perceptions, but a process of reasoning and deliberation about a person's status about which some conclusion, even a tentative or tenuous one, must be made. It is not an academic exercise but a process of decision making that affects the health, lives, and well-being of our patients. Purposeful use of the knowledge and skills of the professional nurse is directed toward the identification of patient strengths and needs, and the formulation of an action plan to achieve the goals that have been established collaboratively by the nurse and patient.

Certainly a goal-directed, rational approach to assessment, in which decisions are made based on knowledge and context, is essential for safe and competent nursing practice. But it also is important to allow and encourage a creative and intuitive approach to identifying and solving patient problems. Ruth–Sahd (1993) argues that intuitive judgment should be acknowledged and developed along with analytic reasoning. "When colleagues question nurses about a patient's status, nurses determine their answers by knowledge, judgment, and intuition. This requires a sound knowledge base as well as a creative imagination" (p. 11). Intuition should be fostered in the novice practitioner to facilitate movement to more expert, purposive practice. Because novice practitioners do not have the benefit of past experience, acknowledging the creative component of knowledge-building allows students to respond to new situations and new patterns of knowing. Intuition depends on cues from the patient; therefore it is holistic and fits into the paradigm of complex problem solving.

Faculty can encourage intuitive reasoning by asking students to include both subjective and objective data when considering patient problems, encouraging creativity and curiosity, sharing their own expert problem-solving and intuitive experiences, and involving students in activities such as case studies and role playing. In addition, they can encourage students to consider how they "feel" about certain patients and clinical situations. The role for the educator, however, must go beyond feelings; educators must facilitate the examination of assumptions, alternative possibilities and explanations, as well as moral and ethical dilemmas. Analytical reasoning certainly is important as nurses proceed with data collection. In addition, however, the data base leads to a list of possible problems (or "hunches"), and nurses must call upon both inductive and deductive reasoning to make decisions about various diagnostic possibilities, develop alternate solutions, and evaluate evidence. It is intuition that leads to critical thinking, as nurses acknowledge their hunches and then seek evidence to validate those hunches. When this occurs, we witness assessment at its highest professional level.

Summary

This discussion has focused on an understanding of the concept of assessment and on the aspects that are integral to the process of assessment in professional nursing practice. It is important that nurse educators consider the totality of assessment and assist students to develop an appreciation of the multiple dimensions of a patient's reality. Teaching strategies, resources, and activities should focus on caring as well as on competent assessment skills, and faculty should encourage reasoning and reflection as they prepare students to deal with the complexity of contemporary society and health care systems. A critical thinking approach is essential to conduct effective assessments and to empower students, nurses, and patients to understand their options and make informed intellectual, professional, and behavioral choices. It is important for nurse educators and students to be committed to the process of discovery and to appreciate that knowledge is necessary not only to answer questions but to ask them. Use of the arts and humanities to help students learn these many dimensions of assessment may facilitate their understanding of the true nature of professional nursing practice, namely, a concern for patients as unique and holistic individuals.

THE ARTS AND HUMANITIES RELATED TO ASSESSMENT

Since the concept of assessment is a holistic one and nurses must assess physical, emotional, social, spiritual, interpersonal, and cultural needs and abilities, the resources available to enhance student learning in this area are numerous. Some examples from sculpture, literature, photography, drama, and film are offered to stimulate ideas of how to teach creatively in this area, but it is important to point out that almost any picture, television show, or film could be used for students to assess people's physical stature, mobility, gait, muscle tone, hair and skin condition, communication patterns, and so on.

Literature

Novels

Part of assessment involves gathering relevant data, organizing and interrelating those data in meaningful ways, and drawing conclusions based on the data. The use of mystery novels can be used to help students develop these skills.[1] *Death in the Air* (Christie, 1965), *Murder on the Orient Express* (Christie, 1960), and *The Mirror Crack'd from Side to Side* (Christie, 1990) are excellent sources for this purpose. All three novels are easy to read, hold the reader's interest, and provide extensive clues and pieces of data about the murder. Students could be told to read one of these books except for the final chapter. After reading the novel, students might be asked to list all the objective and subjective data available to them throughout the book, distinguish relevant from irrelevant data as they pertain to solving the mystery, and draw conclusions about who the murderer is, based on the evidence gathered. After each student has completed this assignment, they could be brought together to discuss their conclusions and the reasoning behind those conclusions. They could then read the final chapter of the book to compare their thinking with that of the person in the book who solves the mystery. This kind of assignment could be fun, introduce an air of excitement, involve some healthy competition among students, and develop important assessment and diagnostic skills, all at the same time.

Many of the books described in chapter 11, also could be used in an assessment course. When reading *Heart Sounds* (Lear, 1980), beginning students could be directed to focus on the "clues" offered by the central figure and his wife regarding his cardiac status, his physical and emotional responses to various treatments, and their ability to cope with the health situation. Similarly, *Bed Number Ten* (Baier & Schomaker, 1985) offers a variety of neurological changes experienced by the main character; beginning

---

1 The authors wish to thank Michelle Ficca, MSN, RN, for this idea. Ms. Ficca uses this assignment with her students in the nursing program at Lycoming College in Williamsport, PA.

students could be asked to document normal and abnormal functioning, formulate nursing diagnoses, make judgments about appropriate interventions, and design a plan of care based on those assessment data.

Poetry

One of the components of assessment that students often find less than interesting is the skin. However, the poem, "Skin," by Marilyn Krysl (Krysl & Watson, 1988, pp. 15–16), which tells how important the skin is, might serve to help students appreciate the significance of a sound skin assessment. Krysl notes that skin is a major organ through which we experience the world around us and we touch other people. Students might be asked to validate the accuracy of the information contained in this poem and use it as the basis for discussion of how to conduct a thorough skin assessment.

Television and Film

The film, *The Elephant Man* (1980), is the true story of a grossly deformed man living in England during the 19th century. He had a twisted spine, a useless right arm, and a head swollen to twice the normal size. Students could, of course, be asked to assess John Merrick's physical status and describe his deformities, gait, respirations, ability to communicate and articulate words, and so on. In addition, however, they could assess how he coped with all his abnormalities: How did they affect his social interactions, cognitive ability, and self-esteem? What strengths did he have, and how did he develop them? How were his sleeping, eating, and elimination habits altered to accommodate his deformities? *The Elephant Man* is an extraordinarily moving story that could serve as an excellent resource to use when helping students develop their assessment and diagnosis skills.

As mentioned earlier, students also might be assigned to watch a variety of television programs to assess the general appearance of characters, their environments, the way they express needs, the kind of support they have available to them, and so on. By having different students watch different programs, they will be exposed to a wide variety of situations that can be compared and contrasted.

Fine Arts

Painting

Paintings could be used to reinforce and evaluate learning of assessment skills, as noted by Loden (1989). This nurse educator organized a one-day clinical experience at a museum of art to reinforce health assessment and nursing diagnosis skills that had been learned by her students. Sophomore students visited the museum to "identify, in works of art, the concept of wellness/illness . . . and to increase skills in assessment" (p. 25). After selecting a single work of art, each student wrote a description of the subject's physical appearance and stage of growth and development; they also had to determine if the subject was healthy or appeared ill, and then justify their conclusion. This experience helped them draw inferences, appreciate the effect of environmental and social conditions on health, and be more observant of clues to define "health," all of which are essential if students are to conduct holistic assessments.

This same idea was used by Davis (1992) with RN–BSN students. Using works on display in her own university's art gallery, Davis selected particular works of art and gave students specific directions to guide their assessments. For example, students were asked to contrast the developmental stages of the individuals appearing in two specific paintings, to identify the health risks in two other works, and to assess the emotional state of the subject in Jerome Within's "Loss of Innocence" based on his nonverbal communication. Again, the experience helped emphasize the extensive amount of data that can be gathered merely through observation, and it helped develop students' assessment skills.

Not everyone, however, has access to a substantive art museum. In that case, the physical form could be assessed using photographs of paintings. "A Ballet Dancer" by Degas, Schignano's "Bust of a Little Boy," Renoir's "Venus Victorious," "Little Dancer Aged 14" by Degas, or "Adam" by Rodin, all present "normal" forms. An abnormal form is presented in Picasso's "Head of a Woman," which could be used to discuss the nurse's immediate reaction to a disfigured individual, documenting abnormalities, and the nature of distortions. Finally, specific aspects of assessment could be tied to certain works of art. For example, students could be asked to do a nursing assessment of the skin of the man and woman portrayed in Beckman's "Double Nude" and include all pertinent objective data. Or after viewing Munch's "The Scream," a stark black-and-white painting of a child in anguish, students might be asked what they would do to calm a child they were to assess, should the child become as distressed as the one in this painting.

Rubens' painting of "Hygeia, Goddess of Health" depicts a woman looking at and feeding a snake. A robe covers her body except for her left breast, shoulder, and arm. This simple painting provides an opportunity for students to assess the full breast, the somewhat large hands, and the muscular, almost male-like arm. Another similar example is "Charity" by del Sarto, which depicts an exposed right breast that is full, an erect nipple, a baby who is at the breast to nurse but has turned away, and two other children in the background. Since breast examination can be uncomfortable for students, the use of works such as these might serve to introduce the topic and provide "safe" subjects to observe and describe using clinical terms.

One of the best-known artists of recent times is Norman Rockwell. His paintings of ordinary, everyday life in America have been seen by millions, and they have adorned the cover of hundreds of issues of *The Saturday Evening Post* for many years. One of Rockwell's paintings, "Be a Man!," shows a thin, bespeckled boy lifting weights as he looks at a poster of a well-developed body builder. Students could be asked to examine the painting, write an assessment of each of the men in it, and then draw comparisons between the two in terms of body structure, muscle development, nutritional status, and other physical elements. They also might be asked to think about each figure's body image and self-concept, providing the rationale for their conclusions in this regard.

Photography

The compelling personal situations depicted by Heiden (1992) in his vivid photo essay of the famine in Africa several years ago provide unique subjects for assessment. Fortunately, most students in this country never see children and adults who are incredibly malnourished, starved and dehydrated, and they may never encounter such individuals in practice. But through the photos provided by Heiden, they can gain an appreciation of concepts like lack of muscle mass, lack of skin turgor, distended abdomens, cachectic features, bulging eyes, protruding joints, and so on. Having seen these dramatic extremes, they have another mental "yardstick" against which to measure the observations they make in practice.

"Types of Emaciation, Aurangabad" by the firm of Raja Deen Dayal was taken to document the effects of malnutrition. The photograph shows approximately 20 children standing together for the picture. In each child, the rib cage is pronounced, all joints are enlarged, eyes and cheeks are sunken, abdomens are distended (to varying degrees), and there is total hair loss. Students viewing this photograph might be asked to describe the physical appearance of the children, assess the physical environment which is apparent, and outline the potential causes for the general appearance of the children. They also might be given an assignment to propose a plan of care—on an individual or community-wide basis—that would address the malnutrition that is evident.

Finally, photographs can be used to expose students to living conditions they might not otherwise see. "Migrant Mother" by Dorothea Lange depicts a pensive mother and the back of the heads of two children; all individuals in this photograph are dirty, and the mother looks tired. Such a picture could be used to initiate a discussion of the life of migrant workers and assess the living, eating, family, and working conditions that would affect the health of all members of a migrant family. Given this kind of understanding and assessment, students could then be asked to formulate appropriate nursing diagnoses and suggest strategies to resolve those problems, strategies that take into account the realities of life of migrant families.

Sculpture

Hoshiko (1985) offered an exiting description of taking students to an art museum to enhance their assessment and diagnostic skills. During a planned field trip and "armed" with specific guidelines, students were invited to wander through the museum and identify various paintings, pieces of sculpture, and other art works that could be used as the subject for assessment. From paintings of 17th century women with exceptionally large breasts, hips and thighs to carvings of a frail malnourished slave, students described what they saw, using "technical" terminology. Hoshiko (1985) noted that one of the most rewarding "finds" was a suit of armor. Upon reflection on this garment and contemplation of the implications of wearing it for any length of time, students formulated nursing diagnoses that related to actual or potential problems with comfort, mobility, elimination, and self-concept. This experience proved to be enjoyable for all involved and provided students with a safe, detached way to look at people, assess their physical status and nonverbal communications, and make clinical diagnoses.

If an art museum is not readily available, however, photographs of various works could be brought into the classroom. For example, "Standing Woman" by Gaston LaChaise is a huge, bronze sculpture of a naked woman. It conveys strength, power, and self-confidence, but it also is an excellent figure to use in helping students develop their assessment skills. Photographs of the statue from all perspectives could be shown to students, and they could be asked to describe the "general appearance," including muscle tone, body proportions, any abnormalities or disfigurements, stance, posture, and so on.

Michelangelo's "David" also could be used in the same way. The one oversized hand on this statue, the muscle development, the unhidden genitalia, and the facial expression all could be used as a common, unchanging human form to be assessed. A discussion on how to describe the abnormality of the hand or what the facial expression conveys would, most likely, reveal different interpretations of what is seen; this could then be used to discuss the need for objectivity, accuracy in reporting, and how the nurse's own biases and perspectives might influence what is observed and recorded.

CONCLUSION

As noted, assessment is the investigation of a patient's situation that encompasses factors affecting health and functioning and that includes the person's perception of his/her strength, risk factors, and problems regarding health and optimal functioning. In light of this definition, there are many opportunities through the arts and humanities to "introduce" students to people of different cultures, health states, and environments. The arts and humanities also allow students to see people "captured in time," as would happen with a photograph or sculpture, or "in action," as would happen with a film or television program. Any of these opportunities can be used to help students develop their observation and listening skills, which are critical to conducting comprehensive and accurate assessments, thereby making the arts and humanities valuable adjuncts to teaching this concept.

REFERENCES

Alfaro–LeFevre, R. (1995). *Critical thinking in nursing: A practical approach.* Philadelphia: Lippincott.

American Nurses Association. (1991). *Standards of clinical nursing practice.* Kansas City, MO: Author.

Baier, S., & Schomaker, M. (1985). *Bed number ten.* Boca Raton, FL: CRC Press, Inc.

Bates, B., Bickley, L., & Hoekelman, R. (1995). *A guide to physical examination and history taking* (6th ed.). Philadelphia: Lippincott.

Benner, P. (1984). *From novice to expert.* Menlo Park, CA: Addison–Wesley.

Burfitt, S., Greiner, D., & Miers, L. (1993). Professional nurse caring as perceived by critically ill patients: A phenomenological study. *American Journal of Critical Care, 2*(6), 489–499.

Calfee, B. E. (1991). Protecting yourself - Nursing negligence. *Nursing 91, 21*(12), 34–39.

Christie, A. (1960, c. 1933). *Murder on the Orient Express.* New York: Dodd, Mead HarperPaperbacks.

Christie, A. (1965, c. 1962). *Death in the air.* New York: Popular Library.

Christie, A. (1990, c. 1962). *The mirror crack'd from side to side.* New York: HarperPaperbacks.

Davis, S. K. (1992). Nursing and the humanities: Health assessment in the art gallery. *Journal of Nursing Education, 31*(2), 93–94.

Ennis, R. (1987). A taxonomy of critical thinking dispositions and abilities. In J. B. Baron & R. J. Sternberg (Eds.), *Teaching thinking skills: Theory and practice* (pp. 9–26). New York: Freeman.

Ford, J., & Profetto–McGrath, J. (1994). A model for critical thinking within the context of curriculum as praxis. *Journal of Nursing Education, 33*(8), 341–344.

Halpern, D. (1984). *Thought and knowledge.* Hillsdale, NJ: Erlbaum.

Heiden, D. (1992). *Dust to dust.* Philadelphia: Temple University Press.

Hoshiko, B. R. (1985). Nursing diagnosis at the art museum. *Nursing Outlook, 33*(1), 32–36.

Jones, S., & Brown, L. (1993). Alternative views on defining critical thinking through the nursing process. *Holistic Nursing Practice, 7*(3), 71–76.

Kozier, B., Erb, G., Blais, K., & Wilkinson, J. (1995). *Fundamentals of nursing: Concepts, process, and practice* (5th ed.). Menlo Park, CA: Addison–Wesley.

Krysl, M., & Watson J. (1988). Existential moments of caring: Facets of nursing and social support. *Advances in Nursing Science, 10*(2), 16–17.

Kurfiss, J. (1988). *Critical thinking: Theory, research, practice, and possibilities* (ASHE–ERIC Higher Education Report No. 2). Washington, DC: Association for the Study of Higher Education.

Lear, M. (1980). *Heart sounds.* New York: Pocket Books.

Leininger, M. (1994). Transcultural nursing education: A worldwide imperative. *Nursing & Health Care, 15*(5), 254–257.

Lindberg, J., Hunter, M., & Kruszewski, A. (1994). *Introduction to nursing: Concepts, issues, and opportunities* (2nd ed.). Philadelphia: Lippincott.

Loden, K. C. (1989). Clinical experience at the museum of art. *Nurse Educator, 13*(3), 25–26.

Ruth–Sahd, L. (1993). A modification of Benner's hierarchy of clinical practice: The development of clinical intuition in the novice trauma nurse. *Holistic Nursing Practice, 7*(3), 8–14.

Stanhope, M., & Lancaster, J. (1988). *Community health nursing* (2nd ed.). St. Louis, MO: Mosby.

7

Caring

Caring is an abstract, complex, and universal phenomenon that is expressed and perceived in different ways across cultures and between individuals. Although the concept is described in the literature and applied in the practice of a number of professions, it is difficult to ascertain a common understanding of the meaning of caring. The considerable attention recently afforded caring within the nursing literature serves to underscore the profession's interest in this concept, as well as the confusion regarding its various conceptualizations (Morse, Bottorf, Neander, & Solberg, 1991). The failure to provide a precise definition of caring is a liability for nursing because it hampers theory development and ultimately affects the applicability of the concept to nursing education, research, and practice. In an attempt to clarify the concept of caring, this discussion includes an explication of its general meaning and a review of how it is described within disciplines related to nursing. The ways in which caring is defined within nursing and, more specifically, nursing education also are addressed. The discussion concludes with a review of specific examples from among the arts and humanities that may be useful to faculty when teaching caring.

DEFINITIONS OF CARING

General Definition

Caring is defined by Mish (1990) as an inflected form of the verb care that encompasses the following meanings: "1a: to feel trouble or anxiety, 1b: to feel interest or concern; 2: to give care; 3a: to have a liking, fondness, or taste; 3b: to have an inclination" (p. 207). This definition expresses a sense of care/caring as an emotion, activity, or attitude in that one feels, has, or can give care.

Definitions Within Related Disciplines

The use of caring as a key term in searching the literature from the social sciences and from philosophy, religion, and education yields numerous references. Many of these, however, address caring from the perspective of its application within a specific discipline and not in terms of its conceptualization. Because of the relatively few articles that offer definitions of caring, one has the sense that the meaning of caring is assumed.

In a discussion of the tension between the caring values and scientific professionalism inherent in the field of social work, Freedberg (1993) suggested a definition of "professional caring" (p. 538) that combines caring with autonomy and knowledge. This author's reflections on caring, as it relates to social workers, are particularly interesting in that the conflicts that are described—for example, society's devaluing of caring as women's work and questions regarding the professional status of social work—are analogous to those experienced by nurses.

Within the context of Freedberg's (1993) model, caring encompasses rational, cognitive characteristics as well as the affective qualities most often associated with the concept. The cognitive aspect underlies the ability of caregivers to recognize their personal autonomy while interacting in a mutual, helping relationship with patients. It is this acknowledgment of self that enables caregivers to respond in a manner that empowers the patient and fosters the growth of both the provider and recipient of care.

Some of the classic discussions of caring are found in psychology literature. Again it is difficult to discern explicit definitions, but characteristics do emerge that have relevance to an understanding of the concept. For example, within the context of therapeutic counseling, there is reference to caring as love. Understanding and acceptance are synonymous with love and are extended by the counselor to the person in need of help (Rogers, 1965). In addition, Fromm (1963) discussed caring as an indication of love and suggested that caring, coupled with knowledge, respect, and responsibility, would foster the integrity and individuality of the giver as well as the recipient of care.

References to the work of both Mayeroff (1965) and Noddings (1984) are found primarily in the literature from the disciplines of philosophy and ethics. The views of both authors also support conceptualizations of caring as described in a number of other disciplines.

Mayeroff (1965) described caring as a human activity that is critical to finding meaning in and experiencing a satisfying life. He asserted that caring occurs between individuals within the context of a developing relationship. The relationship notwithstanding, the participants maintain their own uniqueness and come to a fuller understanding of themselves and the other as individuals. Mayeroff termed this phenomenon of maintaining one's identity within a relationship, "identity-in-difference" (p. 243). He added that if the individuality of the participants is lost, the relationship can no longer be defined as caring. In addition, in Mayeroff's view, providers of care assist others to grow and experience a sense of order in their own lives.

Moral, ethical, and feminist perspectives are integral to Noddings's (1984) view of caring. Noddings addressed caring from the positions of both "the one caring" and "the one cared for" (p. 4). She commented that the critical elements of caring are evident in the interpersonal relationship that exists between the two. The "one caring" is committed to action as a result of an understanding of the "one cared for." Interest in the other is maintained, and the commitment is renewed over the course of the relationship. In turn, the role of the "cared for" is one of "genuine reciprocity" (p. 74).

Kohl (1992) offered a conceptualization of caring from the world view of humanism. He distinguished caring from merely an inclination to act, and described it, instead, as a concern for the welfare of others that is evident in human behavior and actions. Kohl noted that caring enhances human potential. He added that because it also is a rational behavior, caring does not diminish the self-esteem of the recipient or the spirit of the provider.

An understanding of caring, as it is discussed within the discipline of Religious Studies, emerges from an awareness of obligations and ideals that are rooted in various belief systems. For example, Gerken (1991) identified four themes in Matthew's gospel that reflected his understanding of caring. He described these themes as listening, responding, advocating, and hearing, and concluded that providers, as well as recipients, experience healing through participation in caring.

Wuthnow (1991) discussed compassion in terms of caring. In

asserting that caring means "giving of ourselves" (p. 281), he contrasted the concept with the casual performance of social roles and obligations. The author added a caution regarding the need for caregivers to maintain a critical balance between altruism and individualism.

In his article, "On Pedagogical Caring," Hult (1979) provided a conceptualization of caring in the field of education in terms of the student-teacher relationship. He emphasized that pedagogical caring refers to the "carefilled" (p. 243) manner in which teachers perform their roles. Major components of Hult's perspective include the need to know students as persons with rights and worth, the exercise of cognitive and attitudinal behaviors by teachers that reflect caring, and recognition of students as persons with needs and reasonable expectations regarding those needs. In focusing on the student-teacher relationship, Hult noted that the context of the role relationship facilitates teachers' objective appraisal of their own and students' performances.

Definitions Within Nursing

Throughout its history, nursing has been associated closely with caring. In fact, Fry (1988) suggested that the "nature of nursing practice itself" (p. 48) serves as the rationale for the dominant position that caring assumes within the profession. Recently some authors and theorists have described nursing in terms of caring and have posited caring as the essence of the profession (Leininger, 1988; Newman, Sime, & Corcoran-Perry, 1991; Swanson, 1993; Watson, 1988). Regardless of one's personal perceptions regarding the relationship of caring to the nature of nursing, the literature does demonstrate that caring is an important concept in nursing. The implications of accepting caring as integral to nursing are significant in terms of education, research, and practice. Concerns related to such an emphasis are compounded by the lack of critique of the concept in the literature and the confusion regarding its meaning.

In general, the nursing literature reflects a conceptualization of caring that extends beyond the performance of psychomotor skills to a concern for the holistic needs of individuals (Kelly, 1992). Authors also address the undervaluing of caring by society (Reverby, 1987; Roberts, 1990), and describe such behaviors as commitment to and respect for others as critical components of the concept (Koithan, 1994). Additional behaviors identified in the nursing literature as characteristics of caring include assisting others to grow, recognizing the strengths and limitations of individuals, and acknowledging the need for reciprocal caring between nurses and patients (Fry, 1988; Lindberg, Hunter, & Kruszewski, 1994).

Two groups of authors have provided frameworks for organizing the vast amount of nursing literature that addresses caring. Their works facilitate attempts to synthesize the existing perspectives and to move toward clarification of the concept.

Boykin and Schoenhofer (1990) analyzed extant caring theory from five perspectives: "ontological, anthropological, ontical, epistemological, and pedagogical" (p. 149). Their discussion of the essential nature of caring from the ontological perspective is particularly helpful when attempting to define the concept. In reviewing descriptions of caring, Boykin and Schoenhofer identified "authentic presence and connectedness with the other" (p. 150) as common elements. In addition they found that an understanding of caring includes notions of wholeness, being and becoming, and personal and mutual human interactions.

The extensive comparative analysis of explicit definitions of caring found in nursing journals undertaken by Morse et al. (1991) resulted in five conceptualizations: "caring as a human trait, caring as a moral imperative, caring as an affect, caring as an interpersonal interaction, and caring as therapeutic intervention" (p. 122). The five conceptualizations, although not mutually exclusive, do have distinct relevance to nursing based on the definitions, purposes, and outcomes of caring offered within each.

For example, those who define caring as a therapeutic intervention focus on nursing actions that assist patients to achieve their goals. This conceptualization of caring is task-oriented and patient-centered; that is, the knowledge and skills of the nurse are directed toward meeting the identified needs of the patient. The presence of a caring attitude on the part of the nurse is not critical to the achievement of the patient's goals.

In contrast, proponents of the definition of caring as a moral imperative assert that the caring attitude of the nurse is of prime importance. According to this perspective, the ongoing concern that nurses have for patients underlies the decisions they make regarding appropriate nursing actions. Caring, therefore, is the moral foundation of professional practice, and caring behaviors enhance the humanity and dignity of the patient.

A recent quantitative study (Wolf, Giardino, Osborne, & Ambrose, 1994) attempted to capture the essence of caring. The investigators used the term "nurse caring," which they defined as "an interactive and intersubjective process that occurs during moments of shared vulnerability between nurse and patient, and that is both self-and-other-directed" (p. 107). They identified five dimensions of caring through factor analysis of patients' and nurses' responses to the Caring Behaviors Inventory (CBI) (p. 107). The CBI, a 43-item instrument, was generated from 75 items identified in the literature as caring behaviors. The dimensions, "respectful deference to others, assurance of human presence, positive connectedness, professional knowledge and skill, and attentiveness to the other's experiences" (p. 107) serve as empirical referents for the factors that constitute caring and provide a structure for understanding caring situations.

A fuller understanding of the concept of caring in nursing requires that one consider the characteristics of the recipient of care. Nursing acknowledges the person as the primary focus of care. The person is described as an individual, family, or community, at any stage of the life cycle, and at any point along the wellness to illness continuum. In addition, the profession addresses the holistic nature and needs of the person, recognizes and supports the individual's inherent drive toward self-actualization, and emphasizes the uniqueness and dignity of all human beings (Lindberg et al., 1994).

Swanson (1993) commented that designation of the person as the recipient of care also must include the nurse as an individual, as well as all nurses as a group. Her perspective suggests that the commitment of nursing to caring should find expression not only in the nurse-patient relationship, but also in the acknowledgment by nurses of the need to care for themselves and for each other.

Definitions Within Nursing Education

The conclusion of Paterson and Crawford's (1994) analysis of caring in nursing education was that "a clear conceptualization of what caring in nursing education is and how it is transmitted to students does not yet exist" (p. 164). They noted that, in general, reference is made to mutuality and reciprocity in the student-teacher relationship, to the view of caring as both a process and an outcome, and to the assumption that caring empowers students. In addition, Paterson's 1991 study (as cited in Paterson & Crawford, 1994) found that nursing faculty viewed caring as a context for teaching rather than as something that was *done* to students. His review of the literature concluded with an emphasis on the need for research related to how students learn to care as nurses and how nursing faculty learn to care as educators.

The caring curriculum movement provides an impetus for research related to caring in nursing education. This area of inquiry has expanded dramatically in the last decade. Relevant studies were examined recently and categorized according to student-faculty interactions and curricular issues (Frank, 1994). Although much of the research was focused on students' perceptions of caring, Frank was able to identify that students and faculty espoused similar definitions of caring. Common themes that emerged from these definitions were "respect, being present, having competence, and fostering growth" (p. 51). Frank noted that there is a need to investigate faculty perceptions of caring, and for research on the relationship between caring in nursing education and students' abilities to care as nurses.

Analysis of the Various Definitions

Although a common definition did not emerge from this review, an analysis of the multiple definitions of caring identified in the literature did yield several common characteristics. Caring was defined in the dictionary in terms of attitudes and/or actions (Mish, 1990). However, a commonly repeated theme in the definitions offered by many others was that caring requires an attitude of concern that is *reflected in actions* (Boykin & Schoenhofer, 1990; Freedberg, 1993; Hult, 1979; Kohl, 1992; Mayeroff, 1965; Morse et al., 1991; Noddings, 1984; Wolf et al., 1994; Wuthnow, 1991). Thus, a mere inclination to or simply a feeling of caring is not sufficient to describe the concept.

Many authors reflected on the interpersonal aspect of caring, emphasized the mutual and reciprocal nature of caring relationships, and stressed the importance of maintaining the individuality of both the self and the other within the context of a caring situation

(Boykin & Schoenhofer, 1990; Freedberg, 1993; Fromm, 1963; Hult, 1979; Kohl, 1992; Mayeroff, 1965; Morse et al., 1991; Noddings, 1984; Paterson & Crawford, 1994; Wolf et al., 1994; Wuthnow, 1991). Caring, then, is not selfless giving, nor does it foster dependence in the recipient. Instead, caring involves a mutual and reciprocal relationship.

Considerable discussion also has occurred regarding the positive effects of caring on both the provider and the recipient of care. Caring involves mutual growth, fulfillment, empowerment, healing, wholeness, and a sense of connectedness (Boykin & Schoenhofer, 1990; Frank, 1994; Freedberg, 1993; Gerken, 1991; Kohl, 1992; Mayeroff, 1965). Acknowledgment of these positive outcomes supports the notion that caring does not diminish the participants of a caring relationship.

Caring is related to but different from love, compassion, and altruism (Fromm, 1963; Wuthnow, 1991). Mish (1990) listed concern and solicitude as synonyms for caring, but it is difficult to identify similar words that capture the essence of this complex concept.

TEACHING CARING

Bevis and Murray (1990) asserted that "embedded in teaching are the hidden messages about what is valued" (p. 326). They contended that the behavioristic approach, with its strong reliance on lecture and emphasis on the teacher as authority figure, hampers the ability of faculty to teach and students to learn caring. It has been suggested that the capacity to care is developed best in an egalitarian environment that supports dialogue between students and teachers (Bevis, 1993). In such a teaching-learning environment, students and faculty participate actively as learners, share experiences and knowledge, and discuss new ways to find meaning in human experiences.

Although specific strategies to teach caring have not been identified, methods such as role modeling, journaling, reflecting on and sharing personal experiences of caring, and using creative methods such as literature, music, and art have been suggested (Bruderle & Valiga, 1994; Cohen, 1993; Paterson & Crawford, 1994; Watson, 1988). The risk-taking inherent in initiating such strategies cannot be denied, but the benefits in terms of students' ability to think critically, as caring professionals, provide adequate compensation. Perhaps Munhall's (1992) comment will empower those considering the use of creative strategies to teach caring: "We do not want only good performers who can do but participants who can do with care" (p. 371).

THE ARTS AND HUMANITIES IN RELATION TO CARING

Exposure to the arts and humanities puts individuals in touch with who they are as human beings, fosters their understanding of the uniqueness of those around them, and enhances their ability to respond to the needs of others in a sensitive manner. Because the arts and humanities facilitate the development of humanistic qualities, they are particularly useful to foster nursing students' understanding of caring. The works cited in the following discussion were selected for their relevance to caring and for their potential use in teaching the concept.

Literature

Novels

Nursing students' questions related to caring such as, "How much should we care?", and "How will we be able to care for strangers?", are addressed in the novel *Final Payments* (Gordon, 1978). Isabel Moore lived with and provided complete care to her father from the time of his stroke until his death 11 years later. Although her friends said, "You are letting him eat you alive" (p. 6), Isabel believed that the sacrifice of her own life was being done out of love for her father and was, therefore, appropriate and necessary. After his death, Isabel pursued a new life but soon recognized that she had to deal with her feelings about the sacrifices that she had made, and make her "final payments" to the past. Gradually she came to recognize that the rewards of love are the pleasures of life, and that it is possible to help someone without loving them in a personal way.

This well-written novel, full of vivid descriptions and interesting characters, is both sad and humorous. It offers faculty and students the opportunity to reflect on and discuss the nature of caring and the relationship between the provider and the recipient of care. The book also provides a basis for reflection on the need to maintain a balance between helping others and caring for oneself.

Final Payments would be particularly useful as a teaching tool in a postclinical conference. Students could be encouraged to reflect on their current experiences with the expectations of those needing care. Drawing on analogies between their own nurse-patient relationships and Isabel's relationship with her father, students might then share their perspectives on the differences between personal and professional caring.

Currently popularized by its representation as a feature film, the nonfiction book *Schindler's List* (Keneally, 1982) portrays the nature of human compassion in a graphic and emotional manner. During World War II, Oskar Schindler, a Catholic German industrialist, sheltered thousands of Jews and saved them from an otherwise certain death in Hitler's extermination camps. This was accomplished at great risk to himself and with the expenditure of vast amounts of his personal fortune. The themes related to caring that emerge from this work that could be useful to nursing faculty include personal motivations for reaching out to others, the risk-taking inherent in caring, and the moral aspects of the concept.

The inability to care in the truest sense of the concept is described elegantly by Judith Guest (1976) in her novel *Ordinary People*. A mother's denial of her personal needs and feelings after the sudden death of her oldest son in a boating accident renders her incapable of recognizing the needs of her surviving son. As a result she demonstrates care for him by "doing for" as opposed to "being for." In an interesting reversal of stereotyped caring roles, the young man receives support and understanding from his father.

Faculty may find this book useful to initiate a discussion of society's perceptions of caring and the relationship of that to the undervaluing of caring as women's work. In addition, this complex novel offers ideas for discussing the ways in which caring can be demonstrated, and the need for self-knowledge when assuming the caregiver role.

Short Stories

Katherine Mansfield's (1964) *Miss Brill* serves as an excellent example of the short story genre in that it delivers a cogent study of human nature in a few pages. This story of a lonely, elderly woman who partakes of life vicariously from a park bench, is a poignant depiction of the human need for caring and the consequences of not experiencing caring. As the protagonist observes the warm relationship of a young couple in love and longs for that experience in her own life, readers "hear" the often unexpressed needs of individuals for caring. When Miss Brill realizes that the young couple is aware of her presence, she becomes excited about the prospect of being a part of their enjoyment of life. She returns to her apartment feeling rejected when it becomes clear that they are making fun of her.

Miss Brill enables faculty to "set the scene" for a discussion of students' perceptions of how they feel when they do or do not experience caring. The sharing of such descriptions provides insight into the feelings of others and makes one aware of the differences among individuals. It is this awareness that enables nurses to respond to patients' unique needs. In addition, a discussion of how it feels to be cared for can be used to assist students to identify caring and/or noncaring behaviors.

Olsen's (1961) *Tell Me a Riddle* is a short story that explores the demands of caring and the consequences of loss of self through caring for others. For years Eva had cared for her husband and children without regard for her own needs. Her family cannot understand that now, as an elderly woman longing for a life of her own, Eva has nothing else to give. The author provides entry into Eva's thoughts and enables readers to obtain an understanding of her struggle to redefine herself:

> The love—the passion of tending—had risen with the need like a torrent; and . . . drowned and immolated all else. But when the need was done—oh the power that was lost in the painful damming back and drying up of what still surged but had nowhere to go (p. 92).

Bartol (1989) cited this story as an example of a work that enables nurses to understand patients' experiences from an objective perspective. The opportunity to do so emerges from the "aesthetic distance" (p. 456) that literature provides to readers. This story would be useful as students and faculty attempt to construct a definition of caring by distinguishing its critical components. Before undertaking such a task, students could be directed to investigate and bring to class various attributes that might be included in a definition of caring. Group analysis of the suggested attributes could lead to identification of common themes that could then be discussed and debated in terms of their relevance to the concept. Finally, the class can decide whether or not the selfless giving, described in *Tell Me a Riddle*, "fits" with the definition of caring they have constructed.

Children's Stories

The timeless children's book *Charlotte's Web* (White, 1952) emphasizes how one's ability to care for others is influenced by one's past experiences with caring. Thus, it offers insight into caring relationships from the perspectives of the provider as well as the recipient of care (Younger, 1990). In addition, the story addresses self-actualization as an outcome of both being cared for and caring for others.

Charlotte is a spider and Wilbur is a pig. When Charlotte saves Wilbur's life by spinning a message in her web, he struggles to understand her reason for helping him: "Why did you do all this for me? . . . I've never done anything for you." Her response, "I wove my webs for you because I liked you. . . . By helping you, perhaps I was trying to lift up my life a trifle" (p. 164), amazes Wilbur, who had never thought of Charlotte as anything but cruel. Charlotte's caring for Wilbur motivates him to protect her baby spiders after her death, but it is Charlotte whom Wilbur never forgets.

Charlotte's Web could assist beginning nursing students to reflect on why and how they might help others. More advanced students could discuss the book in terms of the nature of caring as they have experienced it in the clinical setting. Questions that could be posed include: "Is caring truly mutual and reciprocal as described in the story?" and "Do patients expect that nurses will care without expecting anything in return?" At even more advanced levels, the book might serve as the impetus for a seminar on the philosophical foundations of nursing and the relationship of caring to the nature of the profession.

The Giving Tree (Silverstein, 1994) is a poignant story about an apple tree and a little boy. The book describes their relationship and concludes with the tree being just a stump, and the boy, tired and elderly. When the tree has nothing left to give the boy other than its stump on which he can rest, it is finally happy. This story might be used to introduce the concept of caring to beginning nursing students. At this level students often ask faculty to discuss how, when, and how much to care, straightforward questions that are not answered easily. An alternative to responding directly to students' questions is to suggest that they use the simple message of this story as a framework for their own reflections on caring, and as an impetus for sharing their various perspectives.

Before reading the story, students might be asked to write their personal definition of caring. They could then read the story and indicate consistency, if any, between their definition and the one suggested by *The Giving Tree*. Faculty could also pose questions to stimulate further discussion such as, "What does caring require of nurses?", "When, if ever, should nurses stop caring?", and "What, if anything, should nurses expect *from* caring?"

The critical relationship between caring and self-actualization is portrayed beautifully in *The Velveteen Rabbit* (Williams, 1975). The rabbit, once the beloved toy of a young child, is discarded with the trash when the child contracts an infectious disease. As the rabbit lies in the heap, he "speaks" to the reader about his search for meaning and what he "sees" as the ultimate futility of self-giving. Rescued by a fairy, the rabbit truly becomes "real" and returns to the garden to watch the child at play.

A number of nursing students may have read *The Velveteen Rabbit* as children. An interesting approach to the book would be to ask students to write their memories of the story and what it meant to them, before reading it from a more mature perspective. This exercise may assist students to recognize developmental differences related to perceptions of caring. The story could also serve as a case study of physical and emotional deprivation. Students, working in groups, could assess the rabbit, identify an appropriate nursing diagnosis, establish goals, and suggest nursing interventions to address the identified problems.

Poetry

"Me and My Work" (Angelou, 1990) provides an opportunity to reflect on the difference between empathy and sympathy. The poem is a man's description of his attempts to support his family, his acknowledgment that others are in more difficult situations, and his plea that he does not want sympathy, which others often confuse with caring.

Because students will need time to consider their responses to this poem, it might be best if faculty read it aloud and allowed several minutes for quiet reflection before beginning discussion of its meaning. An initial question could then be, "What feelings did you experience when you heard this poem?" In order to facilitate students' freedom to express their feelings, faculty should allow the discussion to flow and avoid the urge to comment initially. More specific questions could then follow such as, "How might you respond to this man?" and "What do you think it feels like to be him?" It is important to remember that there are no "right or wrong" answers, and that one of the goals of using poetry is to increase students' awareness of the different ways in which individuals respond to experiences.

Film and Television

The film *Fatso* (1980) portrays the struggles of an overweight man to satisfy his family's demand that he lose weight and conform to their idealized image of him. The story is told as comedy and, indeed, there are many funny scenes. However, the film comes to a poignant conclusion when the protagonist finds acceptance in the eyes of the woman who loves him, just as he is!

The need to examine personal values and to recognize that others' values may be quite different is important to the development of a caring perspective. Because this film addresses acceptance of self and others, it offers salient points for class discussion about caring.

Beaches (1988) traces the lifelong relationship of two women and concludes with the terminal illness and death of one of them. The story takes many emotional turns as the women move apart from each other for a time, and struggle to establish independent, adult lives. Although they develop in completely different ways, they learn that it is their relationship that gives them their greatest strength.

This film evokes many strong emotions; thus, faculty should respect students' need for private expression of feelings if portions are viewed during class time. The mutual and reciprocal nature of caring is a theme in this film that could be explored through class discussion. In addition, students could be directed to identify incidents in the film when one or both of the main characters did not feel cared for, and the impact of that on their physical and emotional well-being.

Fine Arts

Drama

The Man of La Mancha (1965) is a vivid portrayal of the hope and awareness of self-worth that one caring individual can offer another. Aldonza, a woman of the streets, is transformed as a result of Quixote's concern for and interest in her. The woman is unable to fathom this man's love for her because she has never before been "wanted" as a human being with dignity and worth. Quixote, a dreamer who "tilts at windmills," pursues Aldonza and sings of her beauty and value. Eventually, Aldonza sees herself as the reflection of all that Quixote describes and becomes, at last, his Dulcinea.

After seeing this play or even listening to its accompanying sound track, students could be asked to describe their interpretations of Aldonza's transformation and the factors that contributed to it. Students and faculty can learn much by listening to and encouraging each other to share a variety of perspectives. Although all may not agree that caring and being cared for can foster self-actualization, some of the students might be willing to share how they may have grown through the caring behaviors of others. The goal in using the arts and humanities in nursing education is not to build consensus but rather to recognize and respect the differences among individuals.

Students' understanding of the many dimensions of human suffering may be enhanced through reading and discussing Sophocles' ancient tragedy, *Philoctetes* (Jebb, 1984). In this play, Philoctetes, a once-valued Greek soldier, is abandoned on an uninhabited island for 10 years because he has a painful, draining wound on his leg. A young soldier is sent to rescue Philoctetes when his services are required for the army's success in a battle. Believing that his isolation and rejection are about to end, Philoctetes experiences profound betrayal when the soldier must acknowledge that the suffering man is being rescued only for his military ability and not for his worth as a human being. The young soldier's compassionate response to Philoctetes' suffering renews both men physically and emotionally.

In addition to its graphic portrayal of human suffering, *Philoctetes* addresses several themes critical to the education of nursing students. Among its many uses faculty will find the play helpful in discussing, at the introductory level, caring, values clarification, ethical decision making, and society's expectations of nurses. In the clinical setting, the play can facilitate discussion of the "difficult" patient, attitudes of nurses toward patient who are disfigured, and the ability of nurses to respond with compassion to patients with complex needs. Young–Mason (1988) proposed that the play and the characters it presents are useful as analogies for the health care system as well as for care providers. Using her perspective, faculty could assist students to identify and discuss current contexts for the message and moral of *Philoctetes*.

Music

The touching love song from *The Phantom of the Opera* (1987), "All I Ask of You," performed by Michael Crawford, Sarah Brightman, and Steve Barton, raises a significant point about the nature of caring and the expectations of those in need of care. This song could be used as a focal point for a discussion of the characteristics of the nurse-patient relationship and the limitations of human caring. The part of the song where the disfigured Phantom asks the beautiful Christine to love him could be emphasized. Parallels could be drawn between the Phantom and patients who have experienced changes in body image; discussion might then focus on the caring needs of such individuals.

Simon and Garfunkel's "Bridge Over Troubled Water" is a musical recitation of the many things that individuals are willing to provide for each other in a caring relationship. The lyrics of this song convey the importance of support during difficult times and are accompanied by a stirring melody that simultaneously soothes and motivates listeners. This song could be a wonderful way to begin an "Introduction to Nursing" course. After reflecting on the words and responding to the music, students could be asked why they thought faculty chose this song, and what connection it has with nursing. It would be fair to suggest that such an introduction might pique students' interest and assist them to think of the caring dimension of nursing practice in a new way. In later sessions, faculty could refer to this song when discussing the concept of the therapeutic use of self as it relates to caring.

Traditional-age students will, no doubt, be familiar with the song "Trouble Me" by the group 10,000 Maniacs. The lyrics of this song tell of an individual's desire to learn of another's worries and to comfort and support where possible. This song addresses many of the characteristics of caring such as, the need to "know" the other, the interpersonal nature of caring, and the trust required to build a caring relationship. Students could be instructed to choose a line from the song, identify the characteristic of caring that it addresses, and link the characteristic to a patient care situation they have experienced.

Painting

Mary Cassatt's numerous visual interpretations of the mother-child theme offer a rich array of selections from which to choose works depicting caring. "Maternal Caress" shows a young mother with her red-haired baby daughter. The figures are linked by their interlocked arms, and they appear to be concentrating solely on each other. The observer's eyes are drawn immediately to the child's intent gaze on her mother, and to her chubby hand resting on her mother's cheek. This painting could serve as a poignant focal point for a discussion about the affective component of caring. Faculty might ask students to share their views about the differences between caring attitudes, as depicted in the painting, and the actual caring behaviors of nurses. Faculty should allow time for students to "absorb" this work before asking for comments about its meaning.

In Cassatt's "The Bath," a mother is bathing her young child's foot in a basin. The child is leaning on the mother and touching her gently. They both appear engrossed in this intimate activity. This work depicts the "doing" involved with caring and would thus serve as a complement to "Maternal Caress."

Henry Moore, the celebrated British painter and sculptor, depicted the mother-child relationship in a number of his creations. He believed that the mutual caring between mother and child represented the care felt by human beings for each other (Barnes, 1993). "Mother and Child" is a drawing that appears three-dimensional, in that the figures seem to move as one. The young boy is perched on his mother's shoulders; she is holding his left leg and right arm while he touches her face with his left hand. A sense of maternal protection is depicted, as well as the appearance of connectedness between the two.

Faculty may wish to use this work as a way of eliciting students' views of the relationship between maternal caring and nurse caring. The strong message of the mother's support of the child also is a theme in this work that could assist students to understand caring behaviors. Because this visual depiction of one individual literally supporting another "says" so much more about caring than a textbook ever could, students may be more inclined to carry the message over into their relationships with patients.

Sculpture

Maternal caring and human compassion are epitomized in Michelangelo's "Pietà." As Mary holds the dead and mutilated body of her son Jesus in her arms, the marble seems to "come alive" with emotion. Although faculty may need to use a photograph of this sculpture in class, the message of the artist will not be diminished to any great extent. "The Pietà" could function as an alternative to the familiar case study approach in nursing education. After assessing the "family unit" presented in this sculpture, students could identify the level of care needed and plan nursing strategies. This work of art also could be used to sensitize students to compassion, a characteristic so crucial to nurse caring.

CONCLUSION

Although debate about the meaning of caring fosters meaningful dialogue within the profession, competing views affect nursing adversely when they hamper knowledge development. The concept of caring needs further clarification so that its implications for education, research, and practice can be addressed.

Many questions about caring in nursing education remain unanswered. Whether or not caring can or should be taught may be the most significant issue, as the profession struggles to redefine its position in a changing health care system. The examples from among the arts and humanities suggested in this discussion are meant to stimulate faculty members' creativity when exploring this complex concept with students.

REFERENCES

Angelou, M. (1990). Me and my work. In M. Angelou, *I shall not be moved* (p. 12). New York: Bantam.

Barnes, L. (1993, November 24). Themes of Henry Moore. *The Chronicle of Higher Education,* p. B56.

Bartol, G. (1989). Creative literature: An aid to nursing practice. *Nursing & Health Care, 10,* 453–457.

Bevis, E. (1993). All in all it was a pretty good funeral. *Journal of Nursing Education, 32,* 101–105.

Bevis, E., & Murray, J. (1990). The essence of the curriculum revolution: Emancipatory teaching. *Journal of Nursing Education, 29,* 326–331.

Boykin, A., & Schoenhofer, S. (1990). Caring in nursing: An analysis of extant theory. *Nursing Science Quarterly, 3,* 149–155.

Bruderle, E., & Valiga, T. (1994). Integrating the arts and humanities into nursing education. In P. Chinn, & J. Watson (Eds.), *Art & aesthetics in nursing* (pp. 117–144). New York: National League for Nursing.

Cohen, J. (1993). Caring perspectives in nursing education: Liberation, transformation, and meaning. *Journal of Advanced Nursing, 18,* 621–626.

Frank, B. (1994). Caring: Curricular issues. In L. Allen (Ed.), *Review of research in nursing education* (Vol. 6, pp. 33–56). New York: National League for Nursing.

Freedberg, S. (1993). The feminine ethic of care and the professionalization of social work. *Social Work, 38,* 535–540.

Fromm, E. (1963). *The art of loving.* New York: Bantam.

Fry, S. (1988). The ethic of caring: Can it survive in nursing? *Nursing Outlook, 36,* 48.

Gerken, C. (1991). On the art of caring. *The Journal of Pastoral Counseling, 45,* 399–405.

Gordon, M. (1978). *Final payments.* New York: Ballantine.

Guest, J. (1976). *Ordinary people.* New York: Penguin Books.

Hult, R. (1979). On pedagogical caring. *Educational Theory, 29,* 237–243.

Jebb, R. (1984). *The complete plays of Sophocles.* New York: Bantam.

Kelly, L. (1992). *The nursing experience: Trends, challenges, and transitions* (2nd ed.). New York: McGraw–Hill.

Keneally, T. (1982). *Schindler's list.* New York: Simon & Schuster.

Kohl, M. (1992). Humanism and caring for others. *The Humanist, 52*(4), 48.

Koithan, M. (1994). Incorporating multiple modes of awareness in nursing curriculum. In P. Chinn, & J. Watson (Eds.), *Art & aesthetics in nursing* (pp. 145–161). New York: National League for Nursing.

Leininger, M. (Ed.). (1988). *Caring: An essential human need.* Detroit: Wayne State University Press.

Lindberg, J., Hunter, M., & Kruszewski, A. (1994). *Introduction to nursing* (2nd ed.). Philadelphia: Lippincott.

Mansfield, K. (1964). Miss Brill. In K. Mansfield, *Collected stories of Katherine Mansfield.* London: Constable.

Mayeroff, M. (1965). On caring. *International Philosophical Quarterly, 5,* 462–474.

Mish, F. (Ed.). (1990). *Webster's ninth new collegiate dictionary* (9th ed.). Springfield, MA: Merriam–Webster.

Morse, J., Bottorf, J., Neander, W., & Solberg, S. (1991). Comparative analysis of conceptualizations and theories of caring. *Image: Journal of Nursing Scholarship, 23,* 119–126.

Munhall, P. (1992). A new age ism: Beyond a toxic apple. *Nursing & Health Care, 13,* 370–376.

Newman, M., Sime, A., & Corcoran–Perry, S. (1991). The focus of the discipline of nursing. *Advances in Nursing Science, 14*(1), 1–14.

Noddings, N. (1984). *Caring.* Los Angeles: University of California Press.

Olsen, T. (1961). *Tell me a riddle.* New York: Dell Publishing Company.

Paterson, B., & Crawford, M. (1994). Caring in nursing education: An analysis. *Journal of Advanced Nursing, 19,* 164–173.

Reverby, S. (1987). *Ordered to care: The dilemma of American nursing.* New York: Basic Books.

Roberts, J. (1990). Uncovering hidden caring. *Nursing Outlook, 28,* 67–69.

Rogers, C. (1965). *Client centered therapy.* Boston: Houghton Mifflin.

Silverstein, S. (1994). *The giving tree.* New York: Harper Collins.

Swanson, K. (1993). Nursing as informed caring for the well-being of others. *Image: Journal of Nursing Scholarship, 25,* 352–357.

Watson, J. (1988). Human caring as moral context for nursing education. *Nursing & Health Care, 9,* 423–425.

White, E.B. (1952). *Charlotte's web.* New York: Harper & Row.

Williams, M. (1975). *The velveteen rabbit.* New York: Avon.

Wolf, Z., Giardino, E., Osborne, P., & Ambrose, M. (1994). Dimensions of nurse caring. *Image: Journal of Nursing Scholarship, 26,* 107–111.

Wuthnow, R. (1991). *Acts of compassion.* Princeton: Princeton University Press.

Younger, J. (1990). Literary works as a mode of knowing. *Image: Journal of Nursing Scholarship, 22,* 39–43.

Young–Mason, J. (1988). Literature as a mirror to compassion. *Journal of Professional Nursing, 4,* 299–301.

8

Death, Dying, and Loss

Addressing the concepts of grieving, death, dying, loss, and bereavement in the nursing curriculum presents a challenge to educators. Our culture does not talk openly about these subjects, and since they are considered private matters, students typically need a great deal of support as they learn how to discuss grief and loss with patients and families. This situation is complicated by the fact that health care professionals have a tendency to want to save people, cure them, and "make everything better." Death reminds health care professionals that they are not all-powerful, thus adding to the challenge of effectively dealing with this complex concept.

Nursing professionals have made great strides in advocating for dignified deaths, supporting patients and families through the dying and bereavement processes, and meeting the needs of individuals as they face and experience the end of life. In order to be effective in caring for dying and grieving adults and children, nurses need to know how different people conceptualize dying, how patients and families respond to the experience of loss, various social and cultural manifestations of the grief process, and how to assess and meet the nursing needs of grieving individuals and families. Most important, they need to explore and be aware of their own feelings, beliefs, and values about life and death.

THEORIES OF GRIEF

"Grief is the normal reaction to a loss, a universal experience repeatedly encountered. . . . Loss always results in a deprivation of some kind" (Rando, 1984, p. 16). In an effort to understand this universal phenomenon of grief, experts in many fields have studied and reported on it, the results being a variety of theories of grief.

Perhaps one of the earliest attempts to understand the grieving process was undertaken by Bowlby in 1961. As cited in Rando (1984), Bowlby outlined three phases of grief through which individuals pass in dealing with the experience: the urge to recover the lost object, disorganization and despair, and reorganization. Bowlby's work was built upon by Parkes in 1974 (as cited in Rando, 1984) who added an initial phase, that of numbing, where an individual is stunned and denies the loss.

Engel (1964) saw grief as a healing process with several more or less predictable steps. The initial phase, that of shock and disbelief, is followed by a developing awareness, when anger and guilt may occur. The restitution phase includes the funeral and other rituals practiced by the family; those who are grieving then resolve the loss. Finally, the idealization phase occurs, where all negative feelings about the deceased are repressed and the person is idealized; over time, this lessens, and the person is remembered for his/her faults and weaknesses, as well as positive traits.

Another theory that focused on those who are grieving was proposed by Worden (1991), who described four tasks related to grief: accepting the reality of the loss, working through or experiencing the pain of grief, adjusting to an environment in which the deceased is missing, and "emotional[ly] relocat[ing] the deceased and mov[ing] on with life" (p. 16). With this last task, the survivors reinvest their emotional energy in other relationships.

These tasks are similar to those described by Parker and Weiss (1983), although here the acceptance of the loss is not the first task to be completed, as is suggested by Worden's (1991) theory. Instead, Parker and Weiss (1983) note that survivors must first explain the loss intellectually; then they can emotionally accept the loss after repeated confrontations with the reality, and finally assume a new identity. Rando (1984) synthesizes all these theories into the avoidance phase, the confrontation phase, and the reestablishment phase.

In addition to these numerous theories of grief, some of the most significant work related to grieving was done by Elisabeth Kübler-Ross (1969). Her theory of grief was unique in that it was developed inductively, based on interviews she had with dying persons. Additionally, Kübler-Ross's theory offered a unique perspective in that it focused on the person who was dying, not only on those experiencing the loss of that person. Kübler-Ross outlined five stages: denial and isolation (also known as shock), anger, bargaining, depression, and acceptance.

These theories of grief help students understand the phenomenon in an intellectual way. However, the stages, phases, and tasks outlined in each theory suggest that grieving individuals experience these events in a universal, orderly manner. This, of course, is not the case at all. Instead, an individual's reactions to loss are influenced by many factors, including cultural perspectives and personal attitudes.

CULTURAL PERSPECTIVES ON GRIEVING, DEATH, AND LOSS

Death is a universal human experience; however, each culture responds to and deals with it differently. Many cultures see death not as an end, but as a transition from the world we know to one we do not know; in such cultures, individuals are buried with food, ornaments, and personal belongings to make the journey to this new world easier.

Some cultures believe that the dead have power to affect the living; thus, they conduct elaborate rituals, treat the dead person with extraordinary respect, and often call upon him or her. In other societies, the dead are never referred to by name, since speaking a name is seen as an attempt to call a person, and it is believed that the dead person should remain undisturbed. And in some cultures, for example Mexico, symbols of death are very visible in churches, graffiti, ornaments used for decorations, literature, and prominent death notices in newspapers (DeSpelder & Strickland, 1992). Indeed, Mexico celebrates a Day of the Dead festival, during which the dead are honored and families are brought together to celebrate ties with their ancestors.

In essence, then, "each society's response to death is a function of how death fits into its teleological view of life. For all societies there seem to be three general patterns of response: *death-accepting, death-defying,* or *death-denying*" (Rando, 1984, p. 5). In death-accepting cultures, death is seen as a natural part of life, an inevitable event. In death-defying societies, people believe death takes nothing away; it merely puts one in new circumstances or in a new world. And in death-denying societies, such as the United States, death is seen as an unnatural part of human existence, something with which individuals should not have to deal.

It is important for students to learn about the perspectives on death held by peoples of different cultures so that they can be most effective in helping dying and grieving individuals cope with the experience. In addition, they must be well aware of the views of death held by this society and by themselves so that they are careful not to impose those views on others who do not share them.

ATTITUDES TOWARD DEATH

"The study of death is concerned with questions that are rooted at the center of human experience. Thus, the person who sets out to increase his or her knowledge of death and dying is embarking on an exploration that must be in part a journey of personal and experiential discovery" (DeSpelder & Strickland, 1992, p. viii).

Death is an overwhelming experience, whether it is the unexpected death of a high school athlete in an auto accident, the expected but hoped-against death of a severely debilitated woman after major surgery, the long-awaited death of an elderly person with multiple illnesses, or the death of hundreds or thousands of strangers who suffer a natural or man-made disaster in another part of the world. Such experiences overwhelm us because they force us to acknowledge the loss of one or many unique, irreplaceable individuals, they push us to reflect on life and what we have made of our own existence, and they make our own mortality and that of our loved ones only too real.

Ours is a "climate of denial or avoidance" (DeSpelder & Strickland, 1992, p. 6). Many people in the United States try to ignore death's inevitability or construct ways to avoid its reality, and it is thought of as a "bad" thing, a failure, rather than an integral part of human life. However, this is not what the experience of death had always been in this country, nor is it what is experienced throughout the world, as was previously noted.

At the turn of the 20th century in the United States, death usually took place in the home, with family members present. Members of the community shared the grieving process with the family, and death was seen as a natural part of life. But circumstances have changed since then which have led to fewer firsthand experiences with death and greater denial of its existence.

One of the factors that has led to our current attitudes toward death is what has been referred to as "death at a distance"

(DeSpelder & Strickland, 1992, p. 42). As individuals enjoy greater geographic mobility, they move away from family members. There is decreased contact among generations in our culture, and the increase in the nuclear-type family model reduces intergenerational experiences, such as death. Finally, as seriously ill persons are cared for in hospitals and nursing homes, rather than in the home, the dying are segregated from the day-to-day lives of the living.

A change in the importance of religion in our lives also has created a different perspective on death and dying and altered the ways in which individuals reflect on the meaning and purpose of living and dying. In addition, the increasing number and types of technologies available to extend life, lead us to a "whatever can be done should be done" mentality, and encourage us to think about death in more objective, clinical terms (for example, defining death based on physiological indicators) rather than in humanistic, personal terms.

The dramatic rise in average life expectancy and decline in death rates since 1900 have prompted thinking that one can live almost forever, and death is not natural. Additionally, the shift in the cause and nature of death—from being rapid, sudden, and due to acute infectious diseases to being slower and due to more chronic diseases—has led us to think that we can somehow control death.

Finally, the euphemistic language used when referring to dying or death keep it from being a realistic experience. When we talk about people "passing on" or "checking out" or "no longer being with us," we somehow deny the finality or reality that accompanies the words "dying" and "dead."

As a result of these and other cultural phenomena, the attitudes toward death and dying held by many people in the United States make it difficult to talk about this subject. However, if nursing students are to be effective in meeting the needs of the dying and those who are grieving, they must be prepared to confront and discuss death in a realistic manner.

MEETING THE NEEDS OF THE DYING AND GRIEVING

Despite our society's tendency to deny death, nurses and other caregivers often face this life experience. They must be able to form a relationship with the patient and family that conveys caring, compassion, and trust, and use that relationship to make the dying and grieving experience as positive as possible.

One of the first steps in meeting the needs of the dying and grieving is to be honest. Honesty about the illness, the prognosis, one's own feelings, and the values and beliefs of all concerned must prevail if a helping relationship is to evolve. Thus, nursing students must learn to put aside the denial of death and the "taboos" associated with it that characterize our American culture.

Another element in being more effective in meeting the needs of the dying and grieving is to acknowledge that even when one cannot alter the course of an illness or prevent a death, one can still be of great help and comfort to others. Patients and families frequently want to know that someone is there, that someone will listen to their fears and concerns, and that someone is watching out for their best interests. Nurses can fulfill these roles throughout the dying and grieving process; thus, they need not feel impotent, helpless, or powerless, as Smith–Regojo (1995) noted in her reflections of truly "being with" a man as he was dying.

"Everyone who confronts the reality of dying—whether as a patient, family member, or health care professional—needs to experience a supportive environment nurtured by openness, compassion, and sensitive listening" (DeSpelder & Strickland, 1992, p. 142). Elements of such a supportive environment is evidenced in many writings about meeting the needs of the dying; such elements include the right to be treated as a living human being, maintain a sense of hopefulness, not die alone, participate in decisions concerning care, express feelings and emotions, and not be deceived, among others.

In meeting the needs of the dying and grieving, nurses need to help patients and families deal with the many feelings that accompany a terminal illness. Dying persons often feel isolated and separated from all they have known. They and their family members may experience guilt, believing that "If only I had not smoked so much," all would be well. They may worry about the financial burden of the illness and the change it will make in their wage-earning capacity.

Without a doubt, one's self-concept is altered with a terminal illness. Terminally ill persons may see themselves as unattractive due to medical or surgical treatments, burdensome, and unproductive members of society. They experience changes in physical functioning, sexual functioning, and social attractiveness, and they may come to be dependent on others for the most basic functions of life. Thus, caregivers need to treat such individuals with respect and dignity.

In addition to these feelings, dying persons and their families may be extremely fearful. Fear may be related to pain, the expectation of pain, or the worry that pain will not be treated in a timely, effective way. Fear also may center around being abandoned and left alone. Or fear may arise from a concern about not being able to pay one's health care bills and, subsequently, being financially drained. Nurses and other caregivers, therefore, need to be able to recognize the manifestations of fear and institute strategies to avoid, minimize, or help the individual cope with it.

"The terminally ill patient must reorient his life, values, goals, and beliefs to accommodate [the] sudden realization . . . that life, as it has been known, is now limited" (Rando, 1984, p. 199). Throughout this process, the dying struggle for some degree of control. They fear the unknown—that they and their loved ones will experience—and face a great many difficulties, including loneliness, the loss of family and friends, the loss of self-control, the loss of body parts, disability, suffering and pain, the loss of one's identity, regression, mutilation, and sorrow regarding all they will lose.

Finally, dying persons may be discouraged about all they had planned to do with their lives but will no longer be able to achieve. In instances such as these, nurses must find ways to work with the individuals and their families to reexamine life goals and determine ways to meet at least some of them, perhaps in a modified way. For example, a woman may be too ill to actually attend her granddaughter's wedding, but arrangements could be made, perhaps, for the wedding party to stop in to see her on that day and then for her to see a videotape of the wedding afterwards. By being creative and open to all possibilities, nurses can be highly effective in meeting the needs of the dying and grieving.

Nurses caring for individuals who are dying would do well to remember the words of Schulz (cited in Rando, 1984, p. 267): "Of all the needs of the dying patient, the three most crucial are the needs for control of pain, preservation of dignity and self-worth, and love and affection." Students must learn effective ways to help the dying meet these needs.

In addition to helping the dying themselves, nurses have a role to play in assisting those who are grieving, both during the dying process and after the death has occurred. Rando (1984) offers many suggestions for intervening with grievers, although many of her interventions would seem to be appropriate for the dying individual as well.

Rando notes that "what the griever needs most is acceptance and nonjudgmental listening. . . . He will then require assistance in integrating the past with the new present that exists" (1984, p. 79). In order to be accepting and nonjudgmental, nurses need to reach out actively to grievers, and they must be present, physically and emotionally, to give security and support. They need to give grievers "permission" to grieve by encouraging them to express feelings and talk about the deceased, and by not allowing them to remain isolated.

Grievers need to be helped to maintain a realistic perspective throughout the course of their grieving. Acknowledging that each person grieves in unique ways, tolerating volatile reactions, being genuine, realizing and explaining that you cannot make the hurt go away, and not letting your needs prevail all contribute to a realistic perspective.

Finally, caregivers facilitate the grieving process by helping grievers deal with unresolved business, helping them maintain their own health, and helping them develop new roles and relationships.

There is evidence that although they do not become seriously ill or die, most bereaved individuals are at greater risk for a variety of adverse health consequences following bereavement (Committee for the Study of Health Consequences, 1984). Thus, nurses have a responsibility for those who are grieving as well as those who are dying. And since successful bereavement often takes 6 months to a year, nurses will likely need to call upon the resources offered by counselors, support groups, religious organizations, and community groups to help grievers manage the long-term effect of a loss.

ETHICAL ISSUES RELATED TO DYING

Years ago, before technology could be used to repair or replace damaged organs or to keep a person alive seemingly indefinitely, when a person's heart stopped beating and he could no longer breathe on his own, he was pronounced dead. Then came various drugs and respirators which were able to prolong life through artificial means.

Initially, such technological advances were viewed as a boon, and many strove to take advantage of what they could offer. But then the "prolonged life" issue turned into the "right to die" and the "death with dignity" issues, largely as a result of the Karen Ann Quinlan case.

Karen Ann Quinlan was a 21-year-old woman who slipped into a coma due to unknown causes. She was admitted to an intensive care unit and maintained on intravenous feedings and a respirator. After several weeks of remaining unresponsive in a persistent vegetative state with no hope of recovery, Karen's parents asked that the respirator be discontinued so nature could take its course and she could die naturally. The medical staff responsible for Karen's care challenged the parents' decision, and the Superior Court of the State of New Jersey ruled that the medical staff should decide; Karen remained on the respirator. The parents continued to fight for their daughter's right to die with dignity, and they appealed to the New Jersey Supreme Court. Almost one year after her admission, Karen Ann Quinlan's respirator was removed, in accord with the latter court's ruling that the parents should be the decision makers. She was eventually transferred to a nursing home, where she breathed on her own for 10 years before she died, still comatose and still unresponsive.

This case brought to the public's consciousness the many ethical issues that surround death and dying, and it challenged the prevailing goal of "keeping the patient alive at all costs." Ethics committees evolved, Living Wills were drafted, and health care professionals were taught to involve the patient and family in decision making regarding life sustaining treatments. A concern for the *quality* of life came to have as strong a voice as the one for the *quantity*, or length, of life.

In more recent years, "death with dignity," "right to die," and "quality of life" issues have spawned new ethical dilemmas. No longer satisfied with waiting for the inevitable to happen naturally, dying persons and their families have chosen to terminate their lives when they can no longer live fully or when the physical pain or emotional suffering that accompany dying become overwhelming.

We now struggle with distinguishing between ordinary and extraordinary measures to sustain life. We also struggle with the issue of withholding or withdrawing ongoing treatment, including food and fluids. In addition, individuals are asked to sign advanced directives that instruct health care professionals in what to do and not to do under certain emergency or prolonged situations, so that the care providers can act in accord with patients' wishes, wishes that were articulated at a time when they were not in an emergency or particularly stressful situation.

Finally, and even more dramatically, our society now struggles with the issues of assisted suicide and euthanasia. Assisted suicide is the act of providing individuals with the means to take their own life in a painless way, but leaving the actual administration of that method to the individuals themselves. Euthanasia, on the other hand, is the act of bringing about a gentle, painless death. Nurses often find themselves in situations where such actions are being contemplated, and they must be prepared to act appropriately in instances where the dying and grieving processes are "dramatically complicated" (Rando, 1984, p. xi).

THE ARTS AND HUMANITIES RELATED TO DEATH AND DYING

While there are no simple answers to the question of how to help nurses develop the insights, skills, and understanding needed to care for those experiencing loss, the arts and humanities may be particularly helpful in this process. As evident from the preceding discussion, understanding this concept and engaging in effective practice in response to clinical situations involving death and dying requires more attention to the affective domain than the cognitive.

Since increasing one's knowledge of death and dying involves "embarking on an exploration that must be in part a journey of personal and experiential discovery" (DeSpelder & Strickland, 1992, p. xiii), educators would do well to consider teaching and learning strategies that assist in such discovery. Having students read novels and poems, view paintings or pieces of sculpture, or listen to music may do more to increase their self-awareness than would reading a textbook or a clinical journal article; thus, the arts and humanities are particularly useful in helping students learn about the concepts of death and dying.

Literature

Novels

James Agee's *A Death in the Family* (1969), a Pulitzer Prize-winning novel originally published in 1938, is an extremely moving story of a close-knit family that experiences the death of some of its members. First, a grandfather dies of old age and later, Jay, a young man who is married and has two children, dies instantly in an accident at work. The story tells of how the family copes, particularly with the tragedy of Jay, and the changes it makes in their lives. This powerful tale could be used to assess the impact on the survivors of a family tragedy, family coping mechanisms, and how age and circumstances surrounding a death influence people's reactions and abilities to deal with the loss.

Norman Cousins (1979) describes his personal, true-life account of his experience with a life-threatening illness in the book, *Anatomy of an Illness*. This book tells of Cousins receiving a diagnosis in 1964 of ankylosing spondylitis, the poor prognosis that accompanied that diagnosis, and the steps he took to take control of the situation to achieve a positive outcome. In addition to talking about his illness and how he worked to "cure" himself, Cousins talks about the psychology of the seriously ill, which could be used in discussions about death and dying. He notes how patients who were very ill would talk with one another about their fears and concerns, but would not talk about them with health professionals. The feelings of helplessness and powerlessness, the conflict between wanting to be left alone and the "terror of loneliness" (p. 153), the fears of depersonalization and dehumanization, and the lack of self-esteem, all are discussed by Cousins in a personal, powerful way. Although Cousins himself "beat" his disease, his story is a useful one for students to learn about the fears and worries of the seriously ill, and to think about what they, as health care professionals, could do to ameliorate some of those fears, encourage expression of true feelings, and help patients and their families cope with loss.

The tragedy of losing a child is beautifully described in *Death Be Not Proud* (Gunther, 1949), a true story about the life, death, and fighting spirit of a teenager diagnosed with a brain tumor. This incredibly moving story tells of Johnny's courage, determination, fears, intellect, sense of humor, friendships, and loving family, and how they all intertwined during the 15 months of his illness. John Gunther, Johnny's father, was a well-known author and world traveler who enjoyed some degree of power in his life and who was always seeking out new experiences throughout the world, but this personal experience showed him that there are some things we cannot control and that we need to learn to live with that. Although the specifics of treatment for brain tumors have changed in the almost 50 years since this book was written, it is still a poignant tale of one family's experience with the loss of a bright, talented teenager and can be used to convey such understandings.

Children's Stories and Short Stories

A very thoughtful story of life and death has been told in the story of *The Fall of Freddie the Leaf* (Buscaglia, 1982). In this story, Freddie, the leaf, grows from a small sprout in the springtime to a large, strong, beautiful leaf. He is surrounded by hundreds of other leaves whom, he comes to realize, are alike in some ways but very different in others, and he comes to be friends with those leaves on his branch. His best friend helps Freddie think about how a leaf is part of a larger circle of life, how leaves change with the seasons, the uniqueness of each one's experiences, and how leaves die. Freddie expresses his fear of dying, but his wise friend encourages him to think of it merely as another season and to reflect on what he has contributed to others. Through this simple but meaningful story, students are helped to consider the meaning of life and death, the naturalness of death in the circle of life, and how one can face uncertainty without fear.

Blackberries in the Dark (Jukes, 1985) is a more reality-based story that could be used with nursing students. Austin is nine years old when he goes to visit his grandparents for a summer vacation, something he had done regularly in past years. Only now, his grandfather has died since last summer, and visiting the ranch is a sad experience. Austin is withdrawn and does not seem to want to get involved in any activity until he and his grandmother use his grandfather's fishing gear and enjoy an evening of fishing and picking blackberries in the dark. Together they keep their memories of Austin's grandfather alive and celebrate who he had been and all he had taught the young boy. This story could be used in a discussion of children's grief and how to help them grieve successfully. It also could serve to stimulate students to reflect on the people they have known and lost, how they worked through that, what those people had given them during their lifetime, and how both they and Austin may idealize the dead, remembering only the good things.

Jukes (1993) also wrote a most insightful story about a young girl facing the death of her beloved uncle. In *I'll See You in My Dreams*, the young girl and her mother are flying to visit the hospital where the uncle lay dying, and the mother tries to "protect" her daughter from this difficult encounter. But the girl has decided to take action, face the situation "head on," and go through with the visit. The story can be used to gain insight in how children manage death, and it could be used to stimulate a discussion of the ways in which children might be prepared to face the death of a loved one. The story also reminds the reader of the tendency, in this culture, to avoid facing and talking about death, particularly with children; this aspect might prompt a discussion about when and how to tell family members about an impending death, how much to tell children, how families from other cultures might handle the situation, and what the role of the nurse might be when a child will experience a loss.

Goldreich (1977) reports on several other children's books that could be used in discussions of death, dying, and loss, including the following: *The Tenth Good Thing about Barney* (Viorst, 1971), about a young boy whose beloved cat dies; *The Dead Tree* (Tresselt, 1972), which tells how death is a natural part of life; *The Magic Moth* (Lee, 1972), a story of a family's struggle with the slow death of its ten-year-old daughter from a congenital heart defect; and *A Taste of Blackberries* (Smith, 1973), in which a child's best friend dies suddenly after a bee sting. For a class discussion that is to focus on death and loss, each student might be assigned to read one of these stories and report on the insights gained from it. The entire class could then draw on their diverse readings to construct a model depicting the multiple dimensions of the phenomenon of death to illustrate the complexity of this concept. Finally, the class might propose what role the nurse might play in relation to each of those dimensions.

Another short story that conveys the feelings associated with the loss of a loved one is *Letter to My Husband* (Truman, 1987). As the name of the book suggests, the author writes a letter to her husband who died four months ago, although to her it "seems like forty years" (p. 1). She expresses her worry for him—not believing he is totally annihilated and wondering whether he is all right—and the efforts she and the four children have made to go on without him. She reflects on the horrible way he died, her anger, her sorrow, her helplessness, her vivid memories of him, their love for each other, the difficulty in going through his things, and her "uncontrollable grief" (p. 19). As time goes by, she worries that she cannot remember every detail about her husband and then realizes that life goes on and she must be more independent and move in new directions. The many emotions expressed in this short book point out the emotional volatility associated with loss and could help students appreciate how the grieving process evolves over time.

Perhaps one of the best-known and most widely used work of fiction that relates to death and dying is Tolstoy's 1886 short story, *The Death of Ivan Ilyich* (Mack, 1979). This tale tells of the fatal illness of a High Court judge in 19th century Russia, Ivan Ilyich, and the way he reacts to his illness, his impending death, and those around him. This experience leads Ilyich on a journey of self-reflection, looking for some meaning in his illness, and reviewing what he has accomplished and how he has treated others in his lifetime. The person who is Ilyich's only source of comfort and understanding is the butler's assistant, Gerasim, who treats him with compassion, respect, and caring. As noted by Younger (1990) and Young–Mason (1988), this short story can be used to help readers understand the despair and isolation often felt by the dying, the importance of allowing dying patients to reflect on and talk about their life, and the meaning of illness. It is an excellent resource to nurse educators as they help guide students in caring for those who face the end of their life, particularly those who are not happy with what they have done or how they have acted throughout their lives.

Finally, *Is My Sister Dying?* (Young, 1991) is a moving account of a 17-year-old girl who has kidney failure, goes on dialysis, and eventually undergoes a transplant. The story is told by her 14-year-old sister who adores her and eventually—after fighting it in the courts—donates her kidney. In addition to conveying an accurate account of the symptoms of kidney failure, the reactions of all family members to this crisis, the donor process, treatments for this illness, and how patients often "revolt" against all the restrictions placed upon them (by eating potato chips, for example, as the older sister does in this tale), this story offers an excellent portrayal of the worries that individuals have about death. Throughout the story, the younger sister is somewhat neglected in light of her sister's crisis and chronic illness, yet she agonizes over the potential death of her sister. Students reading this story might gain an appreciation of the thoughts that individuals have when they anticipate the death of a loved one. They, then, could reflect on how a nurse might try to encourage a person to identify and express those thoughts and what the nurse could do to help the individual deal with them in a healthy manner.

Poetry

A very moving poem that could help students appreciate the impact of high technology on the process of dying is Joan Neet George's "Grandmother, When Your Child Died." This poem is written by a modern-day mother who "talks" to her grandmother and acknowledges that when the grandmother's child died many, many years ago, the child was at home and was able to be held "through the bitter dawn." But this woman's child "died hard," with a motor beside him and fluids running into his veins, "slipping through the drug-cloud." The visions this poem bring to mind are vivid and real, and it stimulates one to think about the impact on the loved ones when someone, particularly a child, dies amidst so much technology.

The death of a child also is addressed in "For a Child Born Dead" by Jennings (1987). This poem offers the perspective of a parent who laments that not only has the child died, there have been no living experiences by which the child can be remembered and known. It notes the child's "clear refusal of our world" (p. 81) and how pure the parent's grief is. This poem might be used in a class that discusses the experience of stillbirth, how parents cope with such a loss, and what role the nurse can play in helping parents survive the experience. It also might be used to heighten students' awareness of the contextual nature of our world and how people cope with new situations that they cannot put into any "familiar" context or perspective, as was the case for the parent whose ideas are expressed in this poem.

The reaction of a wife and children to the loss of their father is eloquently revealed in "Lament" by Edna St. Vincent Millay (1990). In this poem the mother tells the children that their father is dead but that they and life must go on. In an attempt to keep their father close to them, she promises to make little jackets from his old coats, give his keys to their daughter "to make a pretty noise with," and make use of other things that had been his. She tells them that "life must go on, and the dead be forgotten," but she concludes by saying "I forget just why." In this poem, the mother is saying "the right things" and "being strong" for the children, but she suffers a terrible loss just the same. Perhaps students might be helped to think about how people try to hide their reactions to loss, or that they react overtly in ways that will make others more comfortable while they experience inner turmoil. How a nurse might help people like the mother in this poem also would be an important area for discussion with students.

A very moving poem, written by a nurse, Beverly Eskra (1995, p. 282) is "Ode to a Little Boy." In this poem, Eskra reflects on a little boy who will never know the joy of building sand castles or running in the sun and who has legs but is unable to walk as well as a mouth but is unable to talk. Her words convey the sorrow she experiences regarding this little boy's fate and how caring for him has made her realize that nursing was the right choice for her. Students reading this poem might be asked to reflect on the effect on the nurse of caring for a dying patient and the extent to which the nurse should "get involved" in the situation, a question with which students often struggle.

Perhaps one of the best-known poems about facing death is "Do Not Go Gentle into that Good Night" by Dylan Thomas (1971, pp. 207–218). This poem expressed the wishes of a child that his or her father not simply accept death because he is old; instead, the child begs the father to fight against dying. As technological advances provide more opportunities to prolong and sustain life, it is possible to rage against imminent death and to fight it. In addition, in such instances, the wishes of the dying person sometimes are in conflict with those of the family, as may be the case in this poem. By using "Do Not Go Gentle into that Good Night" with students, nurse educators could initiate discussions of these ethical questions and the nurse's role in meeting the needs of both the dying and the grieving.

On a more practical note, Autry (1991, p. 93) writes about "What Personnel Handbooks Never Tell You." Autry is a manager who is devoted to making the workplace more humane and responsive to the people who are a part of it. In his book, *Love and Profit*, he discusses this concept and includes many poems he has written to express his beliefs. One of those poems helps focus our attention on the impact of a loss, namely, those who have worked with a seriously ill or dying individual. In this poem, Autry acknowledges that, although personnel handbooks describe policies related to funeral leaves, they never give any guidance on dealing with the death of a loved one. Although this is a bit humorous, it does make one think about how widely a loss is often felt and how many people are affected when someone dies. It also may help students realize that the circle of those needing support during times of grieving and dying is not limited to the dying themselves or their immediate family members, but may be considerably larger.

Perhaps the well-known poem "Richard Cory," by Edwin Arlington Robinson (1983), could serve to initiate a discussion of the subject of suicide and our stereotypes of who are the victims of suicide. Richard Cory was a rich, well-dressed, well-educated, highly respected gentleman who shot himself. On the outside, one would think this man had everything to live for, yet he chose to take his own life. Why? What could have led him to such a drastic decision? Students might examine the increasing rates of teen suicide in our society and then speculate on the reasons people contemplate suicide and choose to take their own lives, particularly when they seem to be lacking nothing.

Contemplated suicide also is the focus of Dorothy Parker's "Résumé," (1936, p. 50), although the outcome is quite different from what one might expect. In this short poem, the person considers several means of suicide and decides that living may be the best option. In a discussion of suicide, students might be asked to consider what might be done to help an individual choose to live instead of choose to die, and what the role of the nurse is in that process. Such a discussion might help students reflect on the value of suicide hot lines, the skills needed by those who answer such calls, their own strengths and limitations in dealing with this kind of a situation, and the need for counselors, psychiatric nurse specialists, psychiatrists, and other members of the interdisciplinary team in suicide prevention.

The strength that individuals find when they are faced with overwhelming situations such as death is brought to light in the poem "I Will Live and Survive" by Irina Ratushinskaya (1993). This Russian poetess was imprisoned for several years for challenging the political views of the Communist party. In prison, she faced starvation, bitter cold, torture, humiliation, and death; but her will to live and her belief in her "cause" helped her survive. This poem tells how amidst all that horror she found beauty in a frost-covered window and how that vision gave her strength and courage. Ratushinskaya did not die; she survived her ordeal in that prison camp. But this poem may be a means to help students think about the many ways in which people find the courage to face incredible situations, such as a terminal illness, and how they might talk with a dying person about courage and hope.

Poetry also could be used as a means of expression for students themselves as they encounter death experiences in the clinical area. Schaefer (1995) shared several poems she wrote to help her cope with her father's dying, and these are poems that could be shared with students. Sharing such poems written by others who have experienced a loss or asking students to write their own poems about loss could be used to heighten students' awareness of their own reactions to the death, dying, loss, and grief experienced by their patients and families.

Television and Film

'Night, Mother (1986) is a simple, yet powerful film about suicide that stars Sissy Spacek and Anne Bancroft. Jessie is a divorced young woman who lives with her mother, and who carries on from day to day but with no real purpose. She finally decides, in a most rational way, that suicide is the solution to her situation. The film focuses on the last night of her life when she tries to tell her mother how she feels and why she has decided to take her own life, the mother's refusal to believe her daughter would do such a thing and her attempts to talk Jessie out of her decision, and the interactions between the two women throughout the night. This tragic film provides students with an opportunity to examine the reasons young people choose suicide, discern the signs one might see as clues to a contemplated suicide, and suggest ways one might intervene to help the person explore alternatives other than suicide. One does not walk away from this film untouched; thus, it may be wise to "warn" students in advance about how powerful the film is, allow some time for them to reflect after viewing it, and hold the discussion session about the film immediately afterward, rather than having students view the film on their own and talk about it a week or two later.

The End, a 1978 film starring Burt Reynolds, tells of a man diagnosed with a toxic blood disease and told he has three months to one year to live. It is a poignant comedy about his emotional responses to this diagnosis and prognosis, including making his confession to a very young priest for the first time in 22 years, telling his attorney and best friend that he is going to kill himself, being unable to tell his parents the truth, being able to tell his daughter only that he "will be going away for a while," going to the hospital and asking for the ward where the dying patients are, vowing to die with dignity and all his body parts, wondering what it will be like at the very end, and attempting suicide. This film could serve as a case study for students to analyze in terms of Kübler–Ross's or another theorist's stages of grief and suggest the kind of professional interventions that may be helpful to this man, given his life circumstances and the wishes he expresses in the film about living and dying.

Another film that could be used in the study of death and dying is *Harold and Maude* (1971). Harold is a teenager who lives with his mother in a mansion surrounded by servants. In an effort to gain her serious attention, he fakes approximately 15 suicides; in addition, his only source of fun is attending funerals until he meets Maude, an 80-year-old woman played by Ruth Gordon, who also enjoys attending funerals. Maude's interest in funerals, however, is not morbid the way Harold's is; instead, she attends them because they make her appreciate and reflect on the joys of life. Over time, she helps Harold see that life is worth living and that he can make life whatever he wants it to be. This somewhat humorous film could be used in a study of suicide, factors that lead a young person to consider and attempt it, and how such persons could be helped to think about other alternatives.

The 1989 film, *Steel Magnolias*, features an all-star cast including Sally Field, Dolly Parton, Shirley MacLaine, Daryl Hannah, Olympia Dukakis, and Julia Roberts. It tells the story of a group of strong-willed women living in the South during the 1950s and the personal crises each one faces. One of these women is a diabetic who wants to have a child, but she is told that her life would be in danger were she to go ahead with that decision. She struggles with thinking through the things that are important to her, listens to the advice and threats of those she loves, and decides to have the baby, thereby threatening her own life. This is a moving film that very clearly introduces the role values play in making life-and-death decisions. It is likely to generate a discussion of personal values and beliefs, how to deal with situations when the patient's wishes conflict with those of the family, and how to respect the values of the patient. As such, this film is valuable in the study of death and dying.

In *A Time to Live* (1985), a mother, played by Liza Minelli, helps her young son through the final few months of his life. Throughout this time she is forced to confront her own pain, as well as the pain of her dying son and other members of the family. This film portrays the family's interactions and coping mechanisms and shows the use of denial, blame, and distancing; thus, it provides students with a case study of how a family struggles with the death of a child.

Current ethical dilemmas of who should live and who should die, who receives scarce resources and who does not, and who decides all are evident in the 1957 film *Abandon Ship*, starring Tyrone Power. In this film, Power, the captain of a ship which has sunk, is forced to decide who among the survivors would be placed in the sole lifeboat. This situation forces him to reflect on his values, listen to his conscience, and consider the value placed on different lives. While nurses are not likely to be asked to make such decisions, they often are in the midst of similar dilemmas, and students would benefit from discussing ethical dilemmas related to living and dying before they are intimately involved in such a situation.

Another film that introduces ethical dilemmas associated with dying is *Whose Life Is It Anyway?* (1981), starring Richard Dreyfuss as Ken, a successful young man who becomes a quadriplegic after an automobile accident. The story tells of Ken's reactions to his situation, the decision he chooses to make for himself, and the response of health care providers to that decision. Initially, Ken maintains a light, humorous relationship with those around him, but then he becomes angry and, finally, determined to have some control over what happens to him. He hires an attorney to plead his case to the hospital to discharge him, knowing full well that he will die once he is on his own. He challenges the system by asking, "Why are your rules more important than mine?" and by noting that the cruelty in a situation like his is to remove his option for choice. This very powerful film can be used to engage students in a discussion of patients' rights, autonomy, quality of life, and the role of the nurse in situations where the patient's choice is in conflict with the norms of the system.

Three films made in the 1990s deal with the dying and death of young men from AIDS. In *Long Time Companion* (1990), the 10-year relationship between two lovers is strained by the debilitating illness and the imminent death of one of the partners. Made for television in 1990 and starring Richard Thomas and Sada Thompson, *Andre's Mother* tells the story of the relationship between a homosexual male and his recently deceased lover's mother as both work through their grief. *Silverlake Life: The View From Here* is a "homemade" video documentary of a gay couple that lived together for approximately 22 years. Both partners had AIDS and struggled with the weaknesses, decreased appetite, numerous medications, emaciation, shortness of breath, and other symptoms for years, with one partner finally dying at home, under the care of the other. The film shows the dead body being placed in a body bag and the plans to cremate the body. All three of these films are valuable in helping students understand the reality of death faced by AIDS victims, the impact of the disease and the dying process on the victim's lover, family and friends, and how the relationship between the partners themselves and between the individuals and their families is strained and strengthened by their dying.

Finally, the relationship between a dying person and a professional is depicted in *The Last Best Year*, a television drama. Bernadette Peters plays a woman dying of cancer who is referred to a psychologist, played by Mary Tyler Moore. The psychologist does not want to treat this patient because of unresolved personal feelings related to her father's death, but she does take the case and a relationship develops between the two. It evolves until the patient is not afraid to die, and the counselor cares enough for her to put her own needs aside and let her go. In this film, students can see the stages of grief experienced by both women, the issues a dying person must face, how the health care professional's values can interfere with truly helping a patient grieve, and how an honest, sensitive, open relationship can ease the pain of dying.

Fine Arts

Drama

A 1993 Broadway production, *Angels in America*, is a moving, controversial play about AIDS and our nation's collective conscience about persons with AIDS. It tells the story of a gay couple, one of whom is dying of AIDS, and reveals their anguish and pain. This innovative drama portrays, in a very personal manner, the way this couple experienced grief; thus, its value in bringing this very real situation to life for students is enormous.

Lewis (1977) tells of an instructional drama she created entitled, *A Time to Live and a Time to Die* This play dramatizes "one man's struggle with both the dying process and death itself" (p. 763). It features a man in his 50s who talks about his anguish, isolation, and sense of aloneness. He then interacts with a nurse who is insensitive to his needs and focuses, instead, on mundane tasks or telling him to talk with his physician. The play ends with the man having a cardiac arrest, dying, and being lamented by his wife and daughter. While Lewis provides no information on whether this play is available for performance, it introduces the possibility of having faculty and/or students write their own drama to depict what has been learned about dying, grieving, and the role of the nurse throughout those processes. Through such an exercise, students would be called upon to draw on the literature about theories of grief, consider common reactions to loss, and formulate strategies of appropriate interventions by the nurse.

Painting

"Rachel Weeping" by Charles Wilson Peale presents a very graphic depiction of one woman's reaction to the loss of a child. The child lies peacefully in bed, already prepared for burial, with a fabric strap under her chin to keep her mouth closed and her arms bound straight at her sides. On the bedside stand are numerous forms of medication, apparently ineffective. Rachel looks toward heaven, with tears streaming down her face, obviously distraught. Students could be asked to reflect on what they might say or do were they to walk into a room and find this scene, or to discuss the meaning of a child's death after a long illness.

The grief of parental loss also is evident in several pieces by Käthe Kollwitz, who lost several siblings and a son. In "Überfahren" one sees adults carrying the dead body of a child—one bearing the weight of the body and one gently supporting the child's head—while other children and adults walk along; the pained expressions, bowed heads, and sagging mouths reveal how overwhelming such a loss is and how it affects a wide range of people. "Pietà" depicts an adult clutching the body of a dead child who is lying across his lap; the child has a very peaceful expression on her face, but the adult is obviously distraught, tense, and sad. Finally, "Killed in Action" shows a woman whose face is covered with her hands, obviously in despair, while several small children clutch her dress and look up to her with fearful and pained expressions on their faces. Any of these paintings could be used to stimulate students' thinking about how to help children cope with the loss of a sibling or a parent, how to help the parents or the surviving parent cope with such a loss, and how the loss of a child might affect the relationship between the parents and surviving children.

"After Death" by Theodore Gericault is a vivid portrayal of an old man who has died. The painting shows only the man's head and clearly depicts his sunken eyes, hollow cheeks, partially opened mouth, poor coloring, and the not-so-peaceful expression on his face. Students looking at this painting might be asked to think about the physical effects of a lengthy dying process on an individual and how the person himself, the family and the nurse react to those changes over time, and the meaning of death with dignity.

Music

"In the Living Years" (Mike and the Mechanics) tells about the struggle a grown son endures because he did not have the opportunity for a reconcilation with his father before the father's death. The son feels the pain of not having said the things he should have said long ago. The young man's reflections might stimulate a discussion of the guilt, shame, and remorse families often feel when someone dies, thereby stimulating students to think about the role of the nurse in encouraging families to come together and talk openly during the dying process.

Gustav Mahler's "Kindertotenlieder" ("Songs on the Death of Children") are moving, poignant, and tender expressions of loss. The songs, written in German, reflect the poems of Friedrich Rückert, who had lost two of his own children, and even without understanding the words, the feelings in these pieces are evident. Mahler himself suffered the loss of six of his 12 brothers and sisters to a variety of illnesses, and through this music, one can sense the pain, grief, and lasting effects of loss. Students could be asked to listen to the music and think about the messages it conveys about the grieving process and how one can express grief in many ways.

Sculpture

After experiencing the sudden, unexpected death of her son at birth, Julie Fritsch turned to her skill as a sculptor to find a way to communicate her feelings and her despair. With the support of a counselor, Fritsch created more than 20 figures that revealed her reaction to the loss. Among the pieces are "Anguish of Loss," which shows a nude woman, arms clutched across her chest, sitting on the ground, with head and torso bent almost into a fetal position. "Sharing the Grief" shows a nude man and woman both sitting on the ground, she with her head bent and knees pulled up and he with his arm around her neck and head buried next to hers. Finally, in "Collapsing," the naked woman is seen lying on the ground, with knees pulled up and her head buried in her hands, as if she were sobbing. After viewing these figures, students might be asked to speculate on the relevance of the nudity in these pieces, as well as to reflect on the varied reactions to a loss, the process of grieving and recovery, and how a creative art form, such as sculpting, could be used as a form of healing.

CONCLUSION

The experiences of death, dying, and loss are extremely powerful ones that nurses encounter frequently in their practice. Students can learn specifics of various theories of grief quite easily, but what does not come as easy is learning how to deal with these intense, personal situations. Since the arts and humanities offer so many poignant examples of grief and loss, they would seem to be invaluable in helping students develop a greater awareness of this universal human experience and of how nurses can care most effectively for patients and their families. Integrating a variety of art forms into the teaching of death and dying would seem to be an excellent way of helping students explore and express their personal views, feelings, and values about these life experiences.

REFERENCES

Agee, J. (1969). *A death in the family*. New York: Bantam Books.
Autry, J. A. (1991). *Love and profit*. New York: William Morrow & Co.

Buscaglia, L. (1982). *The fall of Freddie the leaf: A story of life for all ages.* Thorofare, NJ: Charles B. Slack.

Committee for the Study of Health Consequences of the Stress of Bereavement (Institute of Medicine). (1984). *Bereavement: Reactions, consequences, and care.* Washington, DC: National Academy Press.

Cousins, N. (1979). *Anatomy of an illness as perceived by the patient.* New York: W. W. Norton & Co.

DeSpelder, L. A., & Strickland, A. L. (1992). *The last dance: Encountering death and dying* (3rd ed.). Mountain View, CA: Mayfield Publishing Co.

Engel, G. L. (1964). Grief and grieving. *American Journal of Nursing, 64*(9), 93–98.

Eskra, B. (1995) "Ode to a little boy." In C. Sullivan (Ed.), *Reflections of light 1995* (p. 282). Owings Mills, MD: Watermark Press.

Goldreich, G. (1977). What is death? The answers in children's books. *Hastings Center Report, 7*(3), 18–20.

Gunther, J. (1949). *Death be not proud.* New York: Harper & Brothers.

Jennings, E. (1987). "For a child born dead." In I. Linthwaite (Ed.), *Ain't I a woman! A book of women's poetry from around the world* (p. 81). New York: Wings Books.

Jukes, M. (1985). *Blackberries in the dark.* New York: Bullseye Books.

Jukes, M. (1993). *I'll see you in my dreams.* New York: Alfred A. Knopf.

Kübler–Ross, E. (1969). *On death and dying.* New York: Macmillan.

Lee, V. (1972). *The magic moth.* New York: Seabury Press.

Lewis, F. M. (1977). *A time to live and a time to die: An instructional drama. Nursing Outlook, 25*(12), 762–765.

Mack, M. (Ed.). (1979). *The death of Ivan Ilyich.* In M. Mack (Ed.), *The Norton anthology of world masterpieces, Volume 2* (pp. 1084–1131). New York: Norton & Company.

Millay, E. S. (Ed.). (1990). *Collected poems of Edna St. Vincent Millay* (pp. 103–104). New York: Book-Of-The-Month-Club.

Parkes, C. M., & Weiss, R. (1983). *Recovery from bereavement.* New York: Basic Books.

Parker, D. (1936). *The collected poetry of Dorothy Parker.* New York: The Modern Library.

Rando, T. A. (1984). *Grief, dying, and death: Clinical interventions for caregivers.* Champaign, IL: Research Press Co.

Ratushinskaya, I. (1993). "I will live and survive." In I. Linthwaite (Ed.). *Ain't I a woman! A book of women's poetry from around the world* (pp. 141–142). New York: Wings Book.

Robinson, E. A. (1983). "Richard Cory." In G. Gesner (Ed.). *Anthology of American poetry* (pp. 546–547). New York: Avenel Books.

Schaefer, K. M. (1995). Our story. *Holistic Nursing Practice, 9*(3), 11–14.

Smith, D. B. (1973). *Taste of blackberrles*. New York: HarperCollins Child Books.

Smith–Regojo, P. (1995). "Being with" a patient who is dying. *Holistic Nursing Practice, 9*(3), 1–3.

Thomas, D. (1971). "Do Not Go Gentle into that Good Night." In D. Jones (Ed.), *The poems of Dycan Thomas* (pp. 207–208). New York: New Directions.

Tresselt, A. (1972) *The dead tree*. New York: Parents' Magazine Press.

Truman, J. (1987). *Letter to my husband. Notes about mourning and recovery*. New York: Penguin Books.

Viorst, J. (1971), *The tenth good thing about Barney*. Old Tappan, NJ: Atheneum Books Young.

Worden, J. W. (1991). *Grief counseling and grief therapy: A handbook for the mental health practitioner* (2nd ed.). New York: Springer Publishing Co.

Young, A. E. (1991). *Is my sister dying?* Pinellas Park, FL: Willowisp Press.

Younger, J. B. (1990). Literary works as a mode of knowing. *Image: Journal of Nursing Scholarship, 22*(1), 39–43.

Young–Mason, J. (1988). *The Death of Ivan Ilych:* A source for understanding compassion. *Clinical Nurse Specialist, 2*(4), 180–183.

9

Diversity

Nancy C. Sharts–Hopko, PhD, RN, FAAN

The concept of diversity has steadily increased in importance in business and in the delivery of human services throughout the history of the United States. Several watersheds can be identified in the expansion of groups whose human rights are recognized under the law. The emancipation of slaves by President Abraham Lincoln was one. Another was women's achievement of the right to vote in 1920. A third was the recognition of the need for countries to codify and pledge protection of human rights, after the Nuremberg Trials following World War II, in response to atrocities committed by the Germans and Japanese. A fourth was the Civil Rights Movement that began in the 1960s with a focus on race, and evolved into grass-roots movements for equality by women, people with physical or mental disabilities, and sexual minorities.

Men, representing a minority of the population, have dominated business and public affairs since the founding of the United States (Domhoff, 1967). Because of this dominance, the assumption that White, Protestant, middle-class values and lifestyles defined the whole of American culture persisted and was reflected in institutional and government policies. One of the effects of the Civil Rights Movement has been widespread recognition that, in fact, the American population has never been homogeneous (Fishkin, 1995; Tocqueville, 1920).

It has been projected that by the year 2000, the majority of American workers will be people of color (Naisbitt & Aburdene, 1990). Organizational norms that reflect the culture and interests of white males are increasingly inappropriate with a work force that is increasingly non-White and female. Those whose dominance is threatened often react defensively, even pathologically, to maintain the old organizational culture (Schwartz & Sullivan, 1993). The result is that productivity is jeopardized, and many, even most, of the organization's workers and customers are disserved.

With the proliferation of laws to ensure extension of legal rights to all residents, employers and social service providers are struggling to change the ways in which they conduct their business. It is in this context that educators, employers and human service providers strive to understand what diversity means, and how it is to be recognized and affirmed in their institutions.

DIVERSITY AND NURSING

Nurses must be concerned with diversity within their work groups as well as among their clients. People's health beliefs; responses to health threats; acknowledgments of transitions such as birth, puberty and death; definitions of normal family and sexual relationships; responses to people in authority; food preferences; verbal and nonverbal communication styles; and religious practices are among aspects of living that are culturally mediated (Hall, 1976). All are reflected in the way people provide or seek health care; and physical, emotional, or cognitive differences from the norm may impose varying degrees of barriers to people's ability to utilize services or be productive.

At the heart of discussions of diversity is concern about honoring the dignity of all people, about obstacles to people's use of services and about their ability to be productive members of society. Employers and service providers are increasingly required to examine all barriers, both social and physical, and determine what it would take to alleviate or eliminate them. It is increasingly clear that the United States cannot afford to exclude groups of people from educational or employment opportunities for reasons other than their ability to participate. And the cost of environmental modifications that allow for fuller participation are, in fact, often far less than the long-term costs of exclusion (Noble, 1995). The exclusion of groups of people from access to health and social services is contradictory to the very nature of human service and can result in increased morbidity and mortality as well as greater long-term costs of services.

DEFINING DIVERSITY

The American population and organizations within it are pluralistic, that is, inclusive of diverse groups of people. While individuals vary within groups, groups are characterized by a sense of group belonging, or group identity (Blank & Slipp, 1994; Schwartz & Sullivan, 1993). To a varying extent, group members share tendencies, or a culture, including values, beliefs, behavior, and background or experience. Groups may be defined on the basis of such characteristics as ethnicity or nationality, race, religious practice, gender, sexual orientation, age, disability, and family composition.

Diversity of Race

Among physical anthropologists, the concept of race has become irrelevant (Sowell, 1994). Certainly groupings on the basis of skin color, the trend in the 1800s, are meaningless after thousands of years of human migration have blended peoples and cultures.

Yet within health care, it is known that some health risk factors are racially mediated, for example, cystic fibrosis or sickle cell disease. Most peoples other than those of northern European origin have lactose intolerance. There are racial group differences in drug metabolism (Levy, 1993). Socially, too, racial identification has meaning, reflecting a group's shared history and experience. The social marginality of racial minorities results in their disproportionate use of health care services, and their being underrepresented among health professionals (Rosella, Regan–Kubinski, & Albrecht, 1994).

Within broad racial groupings considerable diversity exists. *Hispanic* refers to a commonality of language, not to country of origin or religious homogeneity. *African American* refers to a large group of people who trace their heritage to Africa, but via diverse geographic routes at various times in history. *Asian Americans* can trace their roots to many countries, each with unique cultures, spanning over one third of the globe in both the northern and southern hemispheres. What these groups share is their obvious differentness from the dominant, White population.

Diversity of Gender

Although we may think otherwise, it has been only a brief period in American history that most adult women have been housewives (Gerstel & Gross, 1989; Hochschild, 1989). From colonial times, women participated in cottage industry and small family businesses. Prior to World War II, the economy was primarily agrarian, and women participated fully in the operation of family farms. During the war, some war industries provided on-site child care because the women were so vital to the war effort. It was after the war that, in the booming economy, men returned from the war, women retired from the labor force, and it became possible for them to marry and purchase homes in newly created suburban settings. But women's domestic life was short-lived. By the late 1980s, over half of married women, two thirds of all mothers of children, and over half of mothers of infants were in the workforce (Hochschild, 1989).

Despite the high educational attainment of American women, with over half of undergraduate college students being female, and given an economy that now usually requires two salaries to support a family's middle-class lifestyle, women are still struggling for equality of economic opportunity (Blau & Winkler, 1989; Smith, 1992). Interestingly, Naisbitt and Aburdene (1990) have noted that the qualities of leadership needed to meet current and future challenges in the corporate world are those demonstrated by women. Women already comprise half the workforce, and women are starting businesses at twice the rate of men.

Still, the world of work often functions on the basis of assumptions that favor men and discount the family responsibilities that are still shouldered by women. For example, health and social services and schools still assume that women are available to meet their family members' needs but men are not as readily available.

Diversity of Ethnicity, Culture, and Religious Expression

A shared culture is a shared world view. The way people experience their culture may be likened to the way a fish experiences the fishbowl. That is, the fish does not reflect on his life in water until he is removed from it; that is just the way it is, and he has no need to question it. That it is valid for others to live differently, and that the normative group may have much to learn from ethnic, cultural, or religious minorities, is key to cultural sensitivity.

Intercultural conflict arises when two groups perceive a situation differently and, unable to adequately communicate their perspectives, feel violated (Glazer & Moynihan, 1975). It is not for nothing that Senator Daniel Patrick Moynihan's (1993) recent book on international relations is entitled *Pandaemonium*.

As an example in health care, American nurses taught for many years that it was life threatening to place infants in bed on their backs. Women from various cultural groups rejected this idea, to the consternation of health care providers. Recently the American Academy of Pediatrics identified a connection between positioning infants on their stomach and sudden infant death syndrome, and issued a position paper to that effect.

People often react adversely to persons with foreign accents or dialects (Callen & Gallois, 1987). There is a tendency for members of the dominant group to discount their intelligence. Ethnic minority group members may be categorized in the wrong group. Examples of this include asking Korean clients about life in Japan, or asking Mennonite women if they are Roman Catholic nuns. Sometimes, as in the former case, these mistakes are offensive because of a long history of international conflict and oppression.

That institutional policies and procedures may violate the morality of minority groups, and thus their human dignity, is another central consideration in the concept of diversity. Examples include inflexibility of dietary services, or violation of days of religious observance. Institutions must recognize that ethnic diversity will continue to increase as international travel, study, and work become more accessible, and as world migration continues to increase.

Diversity of Socioeconomic Status

Contrary to popular belief, the United States is not a classless society, though it is possible to move from one stratum to another (Domhoff, 1967). Several occupants of the White House in recent decades illustrate this fact. It is disconcerting, though, for employers to confront poverty within their work force. It may be an expectation that workers buy a certain type of clothing, pay dues to certain organizations, or engage in certain social activities. It is difficult for people to say that they cannot comply with these expectations.

Institutional policies may be biased against clients living in poverty. A clinic serving migrant farm workers may be located several miles from the fields where people with no cars are working. A pediatric clinic may only schedule visits during the day, requiring an employed parent with no benefits to lose a day's pay to seek health care for a sick child. Likewise, a hospital's insistence that parents room in on the pediatric unit penalizes all families in which both parents must work, and especially those with no paid leave. Finally, social services are available only to persons with a mailing address, which presents problems that may seem insurmountable for homeless people.

Diversity of Age

The workforce is aging dramatically, with the post-World War II generation of baby boomers starting to turn 50. In 1976 the average age of American workers was 29; by the year 2000 it is expected to be 39 (Blank & Slipp, 1994). The graying of the labor force is reflected in the nursing profession. Over 20 years ago, it was a realistic expectation that the majority of nurses would have left the workforce within a decade of completing their professional education. Now, however, over half of registered nurses in every age group through age 65 are employed within the nursing profession.

For Americans in their 40s, the age for collection of Social Security benefits has been increased to age 67; current discussions about solvency of Social Security financing include proposals to increase the age to as high as 75 years of age. Paradoxically, though, stereotypes about, discrimination against, and underutilization of older workers create barriers to their productivity (Blank & Slipp, 1994). In reality, it is difficult for employers to be sensitive to the disparate world views and varying needs of older, mid-career and young workers.

Most consumers of health care services are older adults. Beliefs about their capabilities and potential contributions to society color the way in which services are rendered. In addition, physical barriers to transportation to and the use of health care facilities limit older adults' ability to access needed care.

Diversity of Sexual Orientation

Between 2% and 10% of Americans are self-identified gays or lesbians (Nettles–Carlson, 1990). Perspectives on the nature of homosexuality have gradually evolved from a view that it is a deviant, immoral lifestyle choice to the understanding that, in many cases, this sexual orientation is a characteristic with which people are born.

Homosexuality is still stigmatized in American society, as evidenced by the fact that many states still outlaw homosexual activity even among consenting adults, that religious groups struggle with the issue of inclusion of gay and lesbian members, and that discrimination still exists in such arenas as the work place, housing, and child custody. The AIDS epidemic has fueled public aversion to homosexuality. It is relatively uncommon for gay and lesbian workers to "come out" in the workplace (Blank & Slipp, 1994), but secrecy extracts a toll in terms of energy expended on vigilance and erosion of self-esteem.

Gay or lesbian clients may have specific health-related needs that go unmet. Providers' lack of awareness of their gay or lesbian patients and their belief in traditional stereotypes about these people contribute to this problem. Gay and lesbian people may avoid seeking health care, or they may use alternative providers because of their expectation of being treated negatively. It may be difficult for gay or lesbian couples faced with a health crisis to express love and support in a judgmental environment.

Diversity of Physical or Mental Status

Sensitivity to the needs of workers or clients with physical disabilities entails making reasonable adjustments to the physical environment that enable them to be productive or to use services. The Americans with Disabilities Act represents considerable progress in this area, though it is still all too common to see that, for example, the motorized cart rental booth may be located in the middle of a large shopping mall rather than at an entryway.

Some corporations, such as McDonald's, have successfully employed mildly retarded adults for repetitive tasks. Not only do these workers prove to be conscientious, but they take considerable pride in their jobs.

The burden for individuals who have been diagnosed with mental illness is enormous (Kaysen, 1993). Widespread misunderstanding of mental illness results in public fear of these individuals. In the late 1970s, Senator Thomas Eagleton was publicly reduced to tears when the press disclosed his history of depression. The mental health and substance abuse history of Governor Michael Dukakis's wife was hidden from view during his bid for the presidency. It is not unusual to hear speculation about patients whose diagnosis of past or present mental illness is reported during nurses' change of shift. The reality is that many people have achieved excellent control with pharmacologic and behavioral techniques. It is useful to reflect that, well into the 1900s, epilepsy and thyroid disease were viewed as hopeless mental illnesses.

Diversity of Family Structure

From the 1950s until recently, television has tended to present ideal families, typically including a working father, a stay-at-home mother, and several biological children. Two generations of American youngsters grew up with a well-reinforced norm for family structure.

This family ideal did not include employed mothers; divorced, widowed, remarried or never-married parents; foster children; children reared by extended family; multigenerational families; gay or lesbian partners rearing children; or communal families of unrelated persons. In fact, the idealized family represents the minority of families and has throughout most of American history. Before the turn of this century, childbirth claimed the lives of over half of all married women, and blended families were common. The Great Depression saw many families split up by economic hardship.

Even with the well-publicized, high divorce rate among Americans, institutions may react insensitively to employees or clients living in nontraditional families. Clients within the health care system may have a support person whose lack of legal status may preclude that individual being recognized as next of kin. Employees may want to confer dependent benefits on a permanent partner whose status is unrecognized. These are examples of the way nontraditional families are penalized.

DIVERSITY IS *NOT* AFFIRMATIVE ACTION

One of the difficulties employers, educators and providers of human services have is the confusion between the concept of diversity and the related but different concept of affirmative action. Diversity is sensitivity to group identities and needs and to intergroup differences within the population. Affirmative action is a social policy implemented over the last 30 years, and now being reevaluated, to rectify past injustices by making specific minorities eligible for special educational or employment opportunities (Jaschik, 1995; Schlesinger, 1992; Shipler, 1995; West, 1993).

Affirmative action has come under scrutiny primarily because of the difficulty in quantifying fairness, particularly when present efforts are intended to address past injustices. Actual or perceived reverse discrimination has been a problem in workplaces and educational institutions. The abilities of capable minority individuals often have been considered suspect when they were believed to have succeeded because of special treatment.

Diversity refers to recognition that the population comprises many different groupings of people; that all of these groups deserve to be treated with dignity; that few of these groups live in accordance with the world view of White, Protestant males; and that institutions must reflect this reality. Nursing students need to participate in a variety of learning experiences, therefore, that will increase their understanding of the concept of diversity and enhance their acceptance of people and practices that may be different from their own.

THE ARTS AND HUMANITIES IN RELATION TO DIVERSITY

The settings in which professional nurses practice are becoming increasingly more diverse. Thus, faculty in nursing education programs are challenged to provide the cognitive foundation and emotional support that will foster students' development as culturally sensitive persons. The use of selected media from among the arts and humanities provides the opportunity for students to reflect on their own cultural beliefs, develop an accurate understanding of groups and cultures that are different than their own, and explore ways to demonstrate sensitivity to such differences in their personal and professional lives. An in-depth discussion of several specific examples from among the arts and humanities is included in the following section. A list of additional resources that could be used when teaching the concept of diversity is provided at the end of the discussion (see Appendix).

Literature

Novels

The Color Purple (Walker, 1982) is an inspiring novel that spans 40 years in the life of an African American family living in the South. The family's story is told through a series of letters written by a young Black woman. The woman is a survivor, and it is her experiences that challenge and stir the reader's emotions and beliefs. In addition, her candid and realistic descriptions foster an understanding of and empathy with her plight. The book is useful to address such topics as racial differences, oppression, and personal insight.

Insight into the world of California's immigrant Chinese can be gained from the novel, *The Kitchen God's Wife* (Tan, 1991). This compelling story of the life of Winnie Louie provides a detailed account of Chinese history and tradition, as well as the difficulties related to assimilating into a different culture. The story, recounted in the first person, is, in a sense, a gift to Winnie Louie's daughter, Pearl. As Pearl struggles to bridge the cultural gap between her and her mother, the reader is drawn into a life and heritage that truly are unique. Because the descriptions of the treatment of women in Chinese society are quite graphic, faculty should be prepared to address students' feelings about these incidents before discussing the cultural differences, per se.

Although *The Kitchen God's Wife* is somewhat lengthy, it is not difficult to read. Nonetheless, it is unrealistic to think that students could read a number of books of this length during one nursing course. Perhaps faculty could assign this book to one student and similar novels that address different cultures to other students. By sharing their reading experiences with each other, students could have the opportunity to explore a variety of cultures.

Chaim Potok's *The Chosen* (1967) is a sensitive portrayal of Jewish life detailed through the experiences of two fathers and their sons living in Brooklyn. Although it is a simple story, the message of the Jewish experience is profound and unforgettable. Because the families are from different Jewish sects, the book also emphasizes the uniqueness of individuals within groups, and the importance of avoiding stereotypes. Students may be able to identify with the young men's struggles to understand and accept their religious heritage. The book also may help students to recognize that although traditions vary from one culture to another, human experiences are universal, and perhaps, the differences among individuals are not so marked.

Short Stories

The setting of Nadine Gordimer's *Selected Stories* (1983) is her homeland, South Africa. Among the selections are the story of a White woman who thinks she understands racial injustice, a Black student who eschews the White liberals' brand of freedom, and an old Afrikaner who finds himself in an African state under Black rule. Thus, the stories offer insight into racial differences from a variety of perspectives.

Faculty could use the collection as a framework for a debate about opposing views of race. Students could be assigned to read different stories and prepare to defend the point of view described in the reading. This exercise could enhance students' ability to articulate a particular position, and foster their willingness to listen to ideas that are unlike their own.

The premise of Frances FitzGerald's (1986) collection of essays, *Cities on a Hill*, is that "there are real cultural differences in the white middle class" (Degler, 1986, p. 11). To support her contention that these limited differences separate Americans as much as any major differences might, the author explored "four cultural enclaves" (p.11), interviewed the residents, and observed their behaviors. The "cultural enclaves" included the homosexual community in San Francisco; the Reverend Jerry Falwell's church in Virginia; the retirement home, Sun City, in Florida; and the Rajneeshpuram commune in Oregon.

The essays address diversity in terms of age, sexual identity, and religion; and they provide honest, nonjudgmental descriptions of groups the author designates as "eminently American" (p. 11). FitzGerald's perspective on diversity is an interesting one that may expand students' awareness of the differences that *do* exist within groups. It also may help them recognize the importance of coming to know patients as who they are, and not as what they appear to be.

Children's Stories

When Dee Willis's family moves to an all-White suburb, the 12-year-old African American child's life becomes quite difficult. The story, *Hold Fast to Dreams* (Pinkney, 1995) details the challenges that she and her family encounter as they integrate themselves into their new community. With the exception of an English teacher who shares Dee's love of poetry, there is no indication that any members of the White community reach out to the Willis family. The book describes the support that the family members provide to each other, and the dignity, perseverance, and strength through which they survive.

Because this book was written for children, the dialogue is clear and to the point; the message also is clear: Change is never easy, human beings can be very cruel, and family members have to support each other. *Hold Fast to Dreams* also underscores the sense of isolation experienced by people who are different. Perhaps students who have experienced this emotion would be willing to share the circumstances with the group. Students may be surprised to discover that the experience of feeling alone is not uncommon; the differences simply may lie in the factors that created their particular experiences. In addition, the opportunity to relate the experiences of other individuals to personal experiences may expand students' awareness of others, and enhance their ability to demonstrate empathy.

Iggie's House (Blume, 1970) also addresses the theme of integration; however, in this story a White child reaches out to a Black family that has moved into her community. The child, Winnie, accepts the Garber family as being no different than her own, and is confused when the rest of the community does not share her perspective. This children's story could be used to initiate a discussion about the origins of cultural beliefs and prejudices. Students might be willing to reflect on where and how they acquired the values and beliefs that inform their attitudes and behaviors. Perhaps, by acknowledging that their beliefs and values are learned, students might be open to expanding their world views.

Poetry

"Cockroach" (Hoberman, 1985, p. 274) is a children's poem that asks, "Is there nothing to be said about the cockroach which is kind?" After this thought-provoking introduction, the poem describes the many negative emotions directed toward cockroaches, comments on their positive qualities, and concludes with the question, "Is there nothing to be said about the cockroach which is good?" (p. 274). Faculty could use this poem as an analogy to help students explore the basis of their attitudes toward people who are different. A way to begin could be to ask students to think of a group of people who are alienated, discuss the reasons why they think this is the case, and share what they know about this group. Although students may not feel any differently about cockroaches after reading the poem, they may recognize that ignorance often underlies prejudice, and that once the value of an individual or group is acknowledged, prejudices are abandoned.

Film and Television

Commercial filmmakers have addressed diversity from a number of perspectives. *A League of Their Own* (1992), for example, a film about the women's baseball league in the 1940s, explores gender stereotypes and female solidarity. The film raises questions for discussion such as the relationship between women's self-esteem and male approval, and the role of women in the workplace, in the home, and in professional sports. Similarly, *Yentl* (1983) tells the moving story of a young Jewish woman in Eastern Europe who disguises herself as a male to fulfill her dream of becoming educated. Both films emphasize the courage, determination, and perseverance that must characterize oppressed groups if they are going to triumph over seemingly overwhelming odds.

Religious diversity also is the subject of several films. In *Witness* (1985), John Book, a policeman running for his life, finds safety in an Amish community. In order to remain hidden he adopts the ways of the community and dresses in the traditional garb. His attraction for the young Amish widow, Rachel, culminates in their dancing together; an activity that is taboo in Rachel's culture. The two opposing worlds—one violent and one peaceful—coexist for a time, but in the end Book returns to his life in the city, and Rachel remains behind in the shelter of her community. The film is sensitive to the stark differences between the two worlds, and acknowledges, ultimately, that the two can never become one. For this reason it is an excellent vehicle to help students understand the legitimacy of diversity and the need to accept the differences among groups.

The setting of the popular film, *Fiddler on the Roof* (1971), is a small Jewish community in prerevolutionary Russia. The theme is timeless and universal, however, in that the protagonist, Tevye, is in conflict with his daughters who he feels no longer respect the traditions of their faith. In fact, he mourns the daughter who married a Gentile as if she had died, until he realizes that he has to accept the changing times. The film is an accurate portrayal of what it means to be different, and how that difference affects every aspect of life. The scenes in which Tevye talks to God are particularly instructive in that they offer insight into the meaning of the experience from his perspective.

Because *Fiddler on the Roof* is 180 minutes long, faculty will need to preview it and assign selected segments for student viewing. Students may be able to identify with the strong theme of family solidarity in this film. Again, the opportunity to connect information gained from watching the film to personal experiences is especially helpful to the development of empathy and cultural sensitivity. Another important lesson that can be derived from this film is the impact of culture on a person's total being and the need for nurses to consider this when interacting with patients and their families.

It is not difficult to locate films that address the themes of racial and ethnic diversity. Although the selections are numerous, the quality does vary in terms of suitability for educational purposes. Two selections that are of considerable value for use by nursing faculty are *Driving Miss Daisy* (1989) and *Heaven and Earth* (1994).

In the Academy Award-winning film, *Driving Miss Daisy* two individuals, from different racial and religious backgrounds, develop a relationship that spans 25 years. Daisy Werthan is an elderly, wealthy Jew; Hoke Coburn, a Black man in desperate need of a job, becomes her driver against her wishes. They both are members of hated minorities living in a small Southern town and surrounded by bigotry. In the climactic scene of the film, they encounter two Alabama state troopers who seethe with hatred for Miss Daisy and Hoke. Their previous incompatibility vanishes in the face of their shared feelings of anger and helplessness.

This gentle film delivers its quiet message through the relationship that gradually develops between Daisy and Hoke. Their friendship emerges from their willingness to understand themselves, to be open to each other, and to accept the differences that separate them. Because the film puts a very human face on the issue of racial tension, it is particularly useful in nursing education.

Heaven and Earth (1994) is the dramatic saga of LeLy Haslip, in her homeland, Vietnam, and in her new life in the United States.

The film portrays Vietnam first as the beautiful home of quiet peasants and then as a landscape and a civilization destroyed by war. When LeLy marries Army sergeant Steve Butler, she moves to San Diego and lives in her mother-in-law's home. America, viewed from LeLy's perspective is larger than life, with more food than she has seen in her entire life. In her new home, the young woman encounters racism, sexism, her sons' denial of their heritage, and her husband's inability to readjust to life in America. At the end of the film, LeLy makes a return visit to Vietnam to renew her all-important connections with her family and homeland.

Faculty are cautioned that *Heaven and Earth* depicts the Vietnam War in a violent manner. However, the female perspective on the war and its consequences is a critical one. In addition, the film is candid in its representation of America as seen through the eyes of an immigrant from a very different culture. Perhaps, students could reflect on how they might feel if they were LeLy, and what personal strengths they would have drawn on to survive as she did. Because self-knowledge is important to the development of cultural sensitivity, such an exercise could be particularly instructive.

Television programs also have depicted cultural diversity in a variety of ways. Faculty should be careful, however, to avoid programs that stereotype certain cultures and lifestyles. "Roseanne," for example, is a situation comedy that portrays the White working class in America. Although the parents seem to resolve conflicts together, the program, more often than not, panders to stereotypes regarding the role of women, the preference of men for beer and football, and the disrespect of children for their parents. In addition, there appears to be a comedic disdain for those who choose to be different. Faculty could suggest that students identify the stereotypes in *Roseanne* and indicate where and how they may have originated. Armed with an understanding of how such false generalizations become common beliefs, students could propose strategies to dispute such thinking. Unfortunately, they may discover that this is no easy task.

Fine Arts

Drama

The critically acclaimed play, *A Raisin in the Sun*, originally produced on Broadway in 1959, continues to stir the social consciousness of its vast audience. Through the story of a Black family living in Chicago's Southside after World War II, the play speaks to such issues as value systems in the Black family, African American identity, relationships between Black men and women, and generational conflicts in Black communities.

The play is easily accessible in that it has been produced as a film and as a television special. In addition, it is a favorite among regional theater groups and is, thus, often available as a live theater production. Finally, it is brief, and despite its powerful message, not a difficult drama to read. Any one of the incidents in the play could serve as a focal point for discussion of cultural diversity. The statement by Lena Younger, the mother in the story, that "color ain't got nothing to do with it," for example, can be debated on the basis of its accurate depiction of racial differences, and analyzed for its relevance to the hopes and dreams of all human beings.

Music

Paul McCartney and Stevie Wonder tell of an ideal situation in which Blacks and Whites live together in harmony in their song, "Ebony and Ivory." In "Colors of the Wind," from the children's film *Pocahontas*, Vanessa Williams suggests that people who are different are people, too. And on a similar note, the popular children's song, "Small World," suggests that people all around the world have much in common. Faculty could play all three songs for students and ask them to comment on the validity of the themes. Questions that faculty might raise include, "Can individuals come together simply on the basis of their shared humanity?", and "Are there cultural factors and prejudices that prevent individuals from accepting that people are all the same?"

The child in Harry Chapin's song, "Flowers are Red," has an expansive and open view of the world that is stifled by his kindergarten teacher. When he first comes to school he colors things as he sees them, but the teacher informs him that all flowers are red. Finally, he succumbs to her pressure and responds in the same way, namely that all flowers are red. Later, at a new school, the boy meets a teacher who tells him that flowers can be many colors, but he again responds that all flowers are red. The boy's experience points to the impact of learned beliefs on attitudes and behaviors. It also emphasizes how ingrained these beliefs become, and how difficult it is to change them.

Finally, the song, "You've Got to Be Carefully Taught," from the musical, *South Pacific*, comments on the origins of prejudice with lyrics describing how children are taught at a young age to hate those their family hates. Again, this song provides the opportunity for reflection on the origins of prejudice, and can enhance students' awareness of culture as learned beliefs, attitudes, and behaviors.

Painting

Daumier's "The Third Class Carriage" depicts a number of individuals crowded together in a railroad carriage. The two central figures are peasant women, one holding a basket and the other nursing a baby. Other figures include a man in a top hat, and several individuals in business attire. There does not appear to be any social contact between any of the travelers; they simply are unique individuals thrown together by happenstance. This painting could be a metaphor for the human condition: individuals with personal goals and concerns existing side-by-side. Students could be asked to describe the circumstances that unite individuals, and the factors that tend to keep them apart.

Norman Rockwell's painting "Do Unto Others" is an excellent example of the different people who make up our world. The painting shows approximately 20 individuals of all ages and races, both sexes, different cultures, and different religions all standing side by side. Rockwell's inscription across the painting, "Do Unto Others as You Would Have Them Do Unto You," conveys the reciprocity that exists among peoples of the world. Students might be asked to reflect on what some groups, represented in the painting, have "done unto" other groups throughout history and what the effects of those actions have been. They then might be challenged to think about what they have "done unto others"—in obvious and subtle ways—how satisfied they are with those actions, what, if anything, they might like to change, and how they might go about making those changes.

Photography

Photojournalist Robert Freeman's (1993) intent in preparing a photographic tribute to Margaret Walker's poetry collection, *For My People*, was to capture the African American experience in an accurate manner. The pictures are in contrast to the stereotypes that hold that African Americans live in drug-infested ghettoes devoid of values and culture. Because they do portray Freeman's feelings about African Americans, they are an opportunity to explore this culture from a very personal perspective.

CONCLUSION

America truly is a rapidly expanding and ever-changing society. Nursing students need to be prepared to recognize the differences among individuals as well as the similarities that bond them together as human beings. Because cultural differences in terms of gender, race, ethnic background, and religion influence the ability and willingness of individuals to seek and respond to health care, nurses need more than basic knowledge regarding cultural diversity: They need an awareness of what it *means* to be different. Selections from among the arts and humanities provide a humanistic perspective to the understanding of diversity that may enhance students' cultural sensitivity.

REFERENCES

Blank, R., & Slipp, S. (1994). *Voices of diversity*. New York: American Management Association.

Blau, F. D., & Winkler, A. E. (1989). Women in the labor force: An overview. In J. Freeman (Ed.), *Women: A feminist perspective* (4th ed., pp. 265–286). Mountain View, CA: Mayfield Publishing Co.

Blume, J. (1970). *Iggie's house*. New York: Dell.

Callen, V. J., & Gallois, C. (1987). Anglo–Australian's and immigrants' attitudes toward language and accent: A review of the experimental and survey research. *International Migration Review, 21*(1), 48–69.

Degler, C. (1986, October 12). The grouping of America. *The New York Times*, p. 11.

Domhoff, G. W. (1967). *Who rules America?* Englewood Cliffs, NJ: Prentice–Hall.

Fishkin, S. F. (1995). The multiculturalism of "traditional culture." *Chronicle of Higher Education, 41*(26), A48.

FitzGerald, F. (1986). *Cities on a hill*. New York: Simon & Schuster.

Freeman, R. (1993). *Margaret Walker's "For my people": A tribute*. Jackson, MS: University Press of Mississippi.

Gerstel, N., & Gross, H. E. (1989). Women and the American family: Continuity and change. In J. Freeman (Ed.), *Women: A feminist perspective* (4th ed., pp. 89–120). Mountain View, CA: Mayfield Publishing Co.

Glazer, N., & Moynihan, D. P. (1975). *Ethnicity: Theory and experience.* Cambridge, MA.: Harvard University Press.

Gordimer, N. (1983). *Selected stories.* New York: Penguin Books.

Hall, E.T. (1976). *Beyond culture.* Garden City, NY: Anchor.

Hoberman, M. (1985). "Cockroach." In D. Hall (Ed.), *The Oxford book of children's verse in America* (p. 274). New York: Oxford University Press.

Hochschild, A. (1989). *The second shift: Working parents and the revolution at home.* New York: Viking.

Jaschik, S. (1995). Affirmative action under fire. *Chronicle of Higher Education, 41*(26), A22–23,29.

Kaysen, S. (1993). *Girl, interrupted.* New York: Vintage Books.

Levy, R.A. (1993). Ethnic and racial differences in response to medicines: Preserving individualized therapy in managed pharmaceutical programmes. *Pharmaceutical Medicine, 7,* 139–165.

Moynihan, D. P. (1993). *Pandaemonium: Ethnicity in international politics.* New York: Oxford University Press.

Naisbitt, J., & Aburdene, P. (1990). *Megatrends 2000.* New York: William Morrow and Company.

Nettles–Carlson, B. (1990). Gay and lesbian lifestyles. In C.I. Fogel & D. Lauver (Eds.), *Sexual health promotion* (pp. 117–132). Philadelphia: W.B. Saunders.

Noble, B. P. (1995, March 5). A level playing field for just $121. *New York Times,* Section 3, p. 21.

Pinkney, A. (1995). *Hold fast to dreams.* New York: Morrow Junior Books.

Potok, C. (1967). *The chosen.* New York: Fawcett Crest.

Rosella, J. D., Regan–Kubinski, M. J., & Albrecht, S. A. (1994). The need for multicultural diversity among health professionals. *Nursing & Health Care, 15*(5), 242–246.

Schlesinger, A. M. (1992). *The disuniting of America.* New York: W. W. Norton & Co.

Schwartz, R. H., & Sullivan, D. B. (1993). Managing diversity in hospitals. *Health Care Management Review, 18*(2), 51–56.

Shipler, D. K. (1995, March 5). My equal opportunity, your free lunch. *New York Times,* Section 4, p. 1.

Smith, S. G. (1992). *Gender thinking.* Philadelphia: Temple University Press.

Sowell, T. (1994). *Race and culture: A world view.* New York: Basic Books.

Tan, A. (1991). *The kitchen god's wife.* New York: Ivy Books.

Tocqueville, A. de (1920). *Democracy in America* (rev. ed.)(tr. by Henry Reeve). New York: P.F. Collier.

Walker, A. (1982). *The color purple*. New York: Harcourt Brace Jovanovich.

West, C. (1993). *Race matters*. Boston: Beacon Press.

APPENDIX

Diversity of Race

Black Like Me (film, book)
Corina, Corina (film)
Cosby Show (television clips)
Fried Green Tomatoes (film, book)
Glory (film)
Having Our Say (book, play)
In the Heat of the Night (film)
Life on the Color Line: The True Story of a White Boy
    Who Discovered He Was Black (book)
Malcolm X (film)
Race Matters (book)
The Jackie Robinson Story (film)
To Sir, With Love (film)

Diversity of Gender

Adam's Rib (film)
All in the Family (television clips)
Mrs. Doubtfire (film)
Nine to Five (film)
Private Benjamin (film)
The Woman's Room (book)
Tootsie (film)

Diversity of Ethnicity / Culture / Religious Expression

A Man For All Seasons (film)
Crown of Columbus (book)
Diary of Anne Frank (book, film)
Exodus (film, book)
Flower Drum Song (film)
Gandhi (film)

Geisha (book, film)
Love is a Many Splendored Thing (book, film)
Schindler's List (film)
The Disuniting of America (book)
The King and I (film)
The Nine Nations of North America (book)
West Side Story (film)

Diversity of Socioeconomic Status

Coal Miner's Daughter (film)
Pocketful of Miracles (film)
Rachel and Her Children (book)
Tell Them Who I Am (book)
The Good Earth (film, book)
The Grapes of Wrath (film, book)
The Unsinkable Molly Brown (film)

Diversity of Age

Among Friends (book)
Cocoon (film)
Harold and Maude (film)
Mrs. and Mrs. Bridge (film)
On Golden Pond (film)
The Bridges of Madison County (book, film)

Diversity of Sexual Orientation

Advise and Consent (film, book)
Fried Green Tomatoes (film, book)
Serving in Silence (book, film)
St. Elmo's Fire (film)
Tales of the City (book series, film)
And the Band Played On (book, film)

Diversity of Physical or Mental Status

Awakenings (essay, film)
Charlie/Flowers for Algernon (film, book)
Coming Home (film)
Elephant Man (play, film)
Forrest Gump (film, book)
Girl, Interrupted (book)

Harvey (film)
I Never Promised You a Rose Garden (book)
Life Goes On (television clips)
Of Human Bondage (book, film)
Of Mice and Men (book, film)
One Flew Over the Cuckoo's Nest (book, film)
Philadelphia (film)
Rainman (film)
The Famine Within (documentary)
The Miracle Worker (film, book)
Whose Life is it Anyway? (film, play)

Diversity of Family Structure

Bachelor Father (television clips)
Full House (television clips)
Little Man Tate (film)
Ordinary People (film)
Scenes from a Marriage (film)
The Odd Couple (film, television clips)

10

Family Dynamics

Linda Carman Copel, PhD, RN, CS

The family is a dynamic, evolving social system of two or more individuals who are united by blood, affection, or loyalty. Each person is born into a family, and this family serves as the primary influence for navigating the world. The biological, psychological, social, and spiritual influences of the family shape the individual's ability to grow and maneuver through the numerous developmental transitions and problematic situations that arise over the life cycle. The family is the most meaningful group of which a person will ever be a part, and it exerts the most profound and lasting influences over the individual's life. Although most people mature and leave their family of origin or biological family, the imprint of the family beliefs, thoughts, behaviors, and values remain a part of that individual forever.

As people venture into the world and create their own families, a variety of family forms can emerge. The creation of a family form is the result of the diverse ways in which people attempt to meet their personal needs for love and belonging within a group structure. Society, or currently operating social forces, affect the composition of today's families; therefore, it is not uncommon to see such family forms as nuclear families, blended or stepparent families, foster-parent families, single parent families, lesbian or gay families, extended families, and communal families. Freedom to be a part of these diverse family forms has proven to be both satisfying and practical for individuals. In recent years the traditional ways of interpreting the concept of a family have been challenged in the state courts. In 1989 the New York Court of Appeals in a ruling about a homosexual couple's dispute over a rent payment issue, stated that "family" could no longer be defined on the basis of consanguinity (blood ties) or marriage (legal ties). Instead, "family" was delineated on the basis of exclusivity, longevity, emotional commitment, and financial obligation (Janosik & Green, 1992).

As our society becomes more diversified, it is expected that there will be significant changes occurring in the structure of family forms and lifestyles (Aburdene & Naisbitt, 1992). A new and evolving concept of family will emerge as people create the family form needed to provide the nurturing, support, and resources necessary for the health and well-being of individuals, their communities, and their countries. In the future one's family may be simply defined as what the individual declares it to be.

FAMILY FUNCTIONING

An overall purpose of the family unit is to provide continuity and stability, along with a sense of connectedness to others. All people need the support of significant others as they strive to handle ongoing change, meet basic dependency needs, and solve problems. The challenge for the family is to maintain a state of balance while promoting human survival, adaptation, and incorporation of the family members into the larger society. To launch people into the world as productive and responsible citizens, the family must transmit strategies that insure protection, nurturance, socialization, and the transference of social, cultural, and spiritual beliefs and values. Specifically, the parents or adults take the responsibility for accomplishing the family functions. Work is done within the family to teach self-care skills. Family members also must be able to obtain, allocate, and share resources; they must learn how to care for each other, communicate, cooperate, be responsive to the needs of others, and follow rules and social norms. It is the family that provides for the health, education, and spiritual background of its members, and as family members mature, they acquire the knowledge and skills needed to engage in decision making, problem solving, conflict resolution, and dealing with change. With these skills a family can capitalize on its strengths, work to overcome its weaknesses, and use both internal and external supports to respond to stressors.

Accomplishing these major functions is an ongoing task of modern families. A healthy functioning family accepts changing levels of responsibility, negotiates and shifts basic role functions as necessary, and works to adequately handle stressful life situations. Walsh (1993) studied and summarized the characteristics of the functional family. She postulated that the capacity to deal with conflict and overcome adverse conditions without disintegration of the family unit is a growth-producing strategy. The ability to resolve difficulties between the generations without resorting to emotional separation strengthens family integrity. A dyad that can work together to solve its problems, rather than procuring a third person to serve as a buffer against emotional discomfort or help to avoid problematic issues, was viewed as a sign of family health. Maintaining emotional closeness across the generations without blurring the boundaries between the generations or diluting the power of the adult generations develops and preserves positive alliances within the family. In fact, Walsh (1993) noted that when differences between family members are encouraged, creativity is promoted, developmental tasks are accomplished, and personal growth is enhanced. The establishment of a healthy emotional climate is cultivated and valued in a functional family, rather than the family merely doing what is mandated to be right.

A major priority for healthy families is the development of a sense of responsibility that is geared to the developmental age of each person. Adults assist children to develop the ability to negotiate for additional privileges and responsibilities as they mature. Within the couple dyad there is a reasonable balance of emotional expression and use of the intellect for the purpose of attaining the goals of relationship maintenance, nurturance, and appropriate accountability for adult responsibilities. Overall, the family provides the broad context of learning for the individual and fulfills the societal need for procreation and socialization of its members.

Since all families have both strengths and weaknesses, they will inevitably experience stressors that affect their functioning. The severity of the stressors will influence how various family members respond to crisis situations. People react differently to similar situations occurring at different times throughout the life cycle.

Some common dysfunctional behaviors in response to stressors include the overfunctioning of one partner and the underfunctioning of the other partner. Another example of such behavior is the person who distances himself or herself from the family through the use of addictive substances, or by becoming overinvolved in work, leisure, or community activities. Often one partner will do anything to establish and maintain peace in a volatile environment while simultaneously subjugating personal needs and developing symptoms of emotional distress.

In some families a child may be thrust into adult roles or become a substitute parent, taking the place of the absent, ineffective, or unhealthy adult. In other families one or more individuals may lack the coping skills and impulse control commonly used to handle problems and deal with frustrations and unmet needs. These families are at risk for the occurrence of violence within the home. Abuse in any form can occur when people either perceive their situations to be precarious or else feel at a loss for options to help themselves. Power is used to boost self-esteem and establish a sense of control over the environment. As Rollo May (1972) so aptly observed, violence can become the force used to remove that which is seen as a barrier to a person's self-worth or accomplishments. A violent person will attack whoever is accessible, and often this person is a family member. It is an ironic fact of life that people hurt those whom they want to love, and that family situations are the greatest potential source of tension for individuals. As internal and external sources of stress besiege a family, its members often will need support, education, training, or treatment to assist them to effectively manage the distress and the pain that they are experiencing in their lives.

DEVELOPMENTAL STAGES OF FAMILIES

The family life cycle has been conceptualized as a series of developmental stages. The work of Evelyn Duvall (1977), a pioneer and sociologist in the study of families, articulated the developmental transitions that all families make, and the tasks or struggles they encounter at each stage of development. She viewed family development as consisting of two phases: the expanding phase, from marriage until children are raised and leave home; and the contracting phase, which begins when the first child leaves home and ends with the death of a spouse. Table 10.1 lists and briefly defines these identified stages and the basic tasks of each stage.

TABLE 10.1 Summary of Duvall's Eight Developmental Stages of Families and Their Tasks

1. Marriage—the period begins by the joining of families to begin a new family
   Tasks: establishing a marriage and identity as a couple, reformulating relationships in family of origin to include spouse, and making decisions about family planning
2. Early childbearing family—the period begins with the birth of the first child and continues until it is 3 years old
   Tasks: expanding and stabilizing the family unit, integrating the newborn(s) into the family, reconciling conflicts about roles, maintaining the home, accommodating grandparent roles, facilitating the needs of the baby and the parents, especially the marital bond
3. Family with preschool children—the period when the oldest child reaches the age of three until it begins school.
   Tasks: nurturing and socializing children, maintaining a stable marriage, and assisting the parent and child to adjust to separation periods
4. Family with school aged children—the period begins when the first child is 6 or starting elementary school and ends with the beginning of the adolescent period
   Tasks: socializing children, developing peer relationships, promoting school achievement and productivity, maintaining a satisfactory marital relationship
5. Family with teenagers—the period begins when the oldest child turns 13 and ends when it becomes a young adult
   Tasks: balancing freedom and responsibility for the adolescent, maintaining open communication between family members, refocusing on marital and career concerns, and a shifting concern for the welfare of the older generation
6. Launching family—the period when the first child departs from the home and continues until the last child leaves home
   Tasks: releasing children as young adults to establish independent identities, readjusting to new parental roles, reexamining of the marriage relationship, developing new interests beyond parenting, and assisting aging parents
7. Middle-aged family—the period when the last child departs from home and one or both of the couple retires
   Tasks: reestablishing and strengthening the marital relationship, sustaining healthy relationships with children, in-laws, grandchildren,

and aging parents, and handling disabilities and death of the older generation

8. Aging family—the period that starts with retirement and ends with the death of both partners

   Tasks: adjusting to retirement, sustaining individual and couple functioning as aging progresses, accommodating to subtle losses and alterations in income and health, experiencing loneliness, and the death of a spouse or significant others

Source: Duvall, E. (1977). *Marriage and family development* (5th ed.).
Philadelphia: Lippincott.

Other family therapists (Carter & McGoldrick, 1980) proposed a six-stage family development model based on transitions and changes to the family unit, such as divorce, stillbirth, illness events, and natural or person-made disasters. Table 10.2 lists the stages of Carter and McGoldrick's (1980) family life cycle.

TABLE 10.2 Summary of Carter and McGoldrick's Family Life Cycle Model Stages

1. Young unattached adults
2. Creation of a family through marriage
3. Family with young children
4. Family with adolescent children
5. Family launching grown children
6. Family in its later years

Source: Carter, E., & McGoldrick, M. (1980). The family life cycle and family therapy: An overview. In E. Carter & M. McGoldrick (Eds.), *The family life cycle: A framework for family therapy* (pp. 3–28). New York: Gardner Press.

Both frameworks reflect how the various tasks and concerns that arise during the life of a family require the use of negotiation and conflict resolution skills. The potential for problems arises when families are unable to accommodate the changing needs of their members or achieve the developmental tasks of their respective life stages.

Families must teach their members to become interdependent over time to achieve an open structure where movement of people into and out of the family is valued as the norm. Yet, not all members are willing or able to move in and out of their families. Often people will cling to behaviors and ways of thinking that need to be relinquished as they proceed to other stages of development. As a result of these inappropriate behaviors, anxiety is generated, and problems related to entering or departing from the family occur.

THEORETICAL FRAMEWORKS FOR VIEWING THE FAMILY

Research and theory construction on the phenomenon of family began in the late 1940s. One decade later, work with families had gained substantial momentum, and frameworks for viewing family concepts emerged. Some of the theoretical frameworks that significantly expanded the knowledge base about families and influenced clinical practice with families were developmental theory, general systems theory, structural family theory, and communication theory. It is the compilation of the concepts from each of the frameworks, rather than those concepts from a single framework only, that clinicians use to assess family interaction and work with families to facilitate their growth and change.

Developmental Theory

The developmental perspective envisions the movement of the family through chronological stages of development, with each stage introducing tasks for both the individual family members and the family system itself to accomplish. The idea of the family life cycle presents the family as a developmental process where there is growth, adaptation, and evolution of the members from conception until senescence. The family life cycle also is viewed as a series of definitive stages with specified patterns of functioning (Duvall, 1977; Hill & Rodgers, 1964; Rowe, 1966).

In the developmental perspective each family member assumes a position in the family, such as mother, father, or child, and an accompanying set of roles, such as wage earner or caretaker. Each role has identifiable behaviors that are based on the norms of the individual family and the overall society. The successful achievement of the tasks crucial to a particular stage of development prepares people for accomplishing later tasks and obtaining society's approval. This framework captures the history of the family as members interact with one another; it recognizes critical events in the individual's and family's development; and it allows a clinician to predict or hypothesize the challenges facing a family at a specific point in its life cycle. The use of the developmental perspective to understand families is believed by some authors (Gillis, Highley, Roberts, & Martinson, 1989; Rowe, 1966) to be limited to the traditional nuclear family, because it does not readily apply to all family forms found in the current social milieu.

Family Systems Theory

Murray Bowen was a major proponent of family systems theory. He viewed the family as a multigenerational system characterized by emotional interaction patterns that cause emotional illness (Bowen, 1978). Members of families struggle with developing and maintaining a positive sense of self and behaviors that are personally chosen rather than based on the power and influence of others. Bowen (1978) believed that emotionally impaired people would base their lives on their emotions and be unable to distinguish facts from feelings. According to Bowen (1978), the degree to which a person is able to define the self as being distinct from others is called differentiation. People with a high level of differentiation are able to separate thoughts from feelings, do not allow feelings to color their thinking process, and can modify their positions as they are exposed to new information. People with low differentiation would have their behaviors dominated by their feelings and be preoccupied with seeking approval from others.

Bowen (1978) described the two-person system within the family as unstable and having the tendency to pull in another person, object, or issue to create stability. The creation of the "emotional triangle" occurs when both anxiety and a low level of differentiation are present within the dyad. A triangle prevents people from dealing with the conflictual situation by allowing them to focus on anything but the issue at hand. Typical examples of "triangles" are a child's acting-out behavior; an adult's overinvolvement with groups, religion, work, sleep, depression, sex; or the development of illness.

The family projection process describes the manner in which the lack of differentiation of the parents is directed at the children. When parental problems become focused on one or more children, the results are an emotional triangle, typically a mother-father-child triangle. Emotional impairment of the child is manifested by a high level of anxiety and subsequent behavior problems. In times of severe family stress, the family will manage the anxiety not only through the use of projection onto children, but also with emotional distance, marital conflict, or the physical, emotional, or social dysfunction of one partner.

Every family has a multigenerational transmission process which encompasses the patterns of interaction that are passed from one generation to the next. Each generation is linked to past and future generations through family relationships. The norms, values, beliefs, behaviors, problems, issues, and patterns of relationships are transmitted from one generation to another.

Bowen (1978) asserted that sibling position, or the place and role one assumes in a family, established by birth order and gender, will have an impact on future adult behavior. The work of Walter Toman (1969) supported Bowen's notion that sibling position and family configurations predict personality traits and behaviors. Sibling position also is predictive of whether a person will take on an overfunctioning or underfunctioning role.

Families are influenced by the way their members leave their primary family. Bowen (1978) conjectured that the way people separate from their family of origin reflects their level of differentiation. Becoming physically or emotionally separated from one's family through an emotional cutoff, is a dysfunctional response and indicates a low level of differentiation.

Systems theory has been used to study both expanding and contracting families, families in stress, and families as open systems (Fawcett, 1977; Gillis et al., 1989; Holaday, 1981; Knafl & Deatrick, 1987; Olson, Sprenkle, & Russell 1979; Smith, 1983). This model is useful for studying various dimensions of the family and its functioning.

Structural Theory

A structural theory for working with families was developed by Minuchin, Montalvo, Guerney, Rosman, and Schumer (1967). It postulated that the family is the basic social system through which people learn to conduct and express themselves. The family structure provides the regulating codes that people use to carry out the activities of daily life necessary for survival and growth. Individual behavior is a product of the structure and organization of the family, as well as of the patterns of interactions among family members.

In the family structural model, the family is viewed as a set of subsystems within the larger family unit. Usually parents, spouses, siblings, and grandparents are defined as subsystems. Each subsystem needs clear boundaries to secure itself from encroachment by other subsystems, and to promote emotional connectedness among its members. Boundaries function to maintain the separation of one subsystem from another. Often a major characteristic of a dysfunctional family is the problems noted with boundaries. Minuchin, Rosman and Baker (1978) felt that families with rigid boundaries had inhibited interactions and produced emotional isolation. Conversely, they noted that overinvolved families had diffuse boundaries characterized by extremely intense, emotionally charged interactions, and power conflicts.

Alignment, defined as the joining or opposition of family members with each other, is another concept in the family structural model that explains how the family system is operating (Aponte & Van Deusen, 1981). The last concept, power, is described as the influence of each family member on the others. Power is evident when one person directs or dictates how things will happen, or when one prevails over others in times of disagreement.

The structural approach to families has been widely used by practitioners and researchers with families whose members have chronic illnesses, or problems with addiction (Minuchin et al., 1967, 1978; Stanton & Todd, 1979). Clinicians use the structural model for constructing and reorganizing families in order to assist them with achieving change.

Communication Theory

Communication theory focuses on the patterns of communication in families. Emphasis is placed on nonverbal interactions and assisting people to recognize that problems in the family are related to unclear communication among its members (Satir, 1982; Weakland, 1976). Satir (1972) asserted that the exchange of information within the family occurs in predictable, repetitive patterns, and there are both spoken and unspoken rules about issues that can and cannot be discussed in families. As is the case in all aspects of life, the message sent by one member of a family is not necessarily the same message received by other family members, or sometimes the message sent is followed by a second message that contradicts the first. This is called double-bind communication, and it commonly occurs in dysfunctional families. Factors that impact on how people communicate are power, emotions, and cognitions (Satir, Stachwiak, & Taschmen, 1977). The major premise underlying effective communication is the self-concept of each family member; relationships are strong and functional when people have adequate self-esteem.

Communication theory is used widely by clinicians who explore and analyze family communication patterns. The content of communication and how it is shared with others, as well as the process or feelings behind what is conveyed are important data to assess the health of families (Satir, 1972; Watzlawick, Beavin, & Jackson, 1967; Wynne, 1978). Methods of communication used in family transactions are directly related to the family's health and well-being.

The above sampling of some of the theoretical frameworks used to understand families is still in need of continued refinement. Further gathering of empirical data will provide evidence to support or refute the conceptual formulations of each model and thereby contribute to future theory development. Today, practitioners and researchers often use integrated models as their frameworks for assessing and intervening in the promotion of family health and the alleviation of dysfunctional behaviors.

FAMILY STRENGTHS AND BEHAVIORS

Families produce the greatest sources of love and the greatest potential for stress. All families exhibit strengths and weaknesses. Over the years, practitioners (Barnhill, 1979; Curran, 1983; Lewis, Beavers, Gossett, & Phillips 1976; Stinnett & DeFrain, 1985) have directed their energies toward identifying and building family strengths as a means to promote family health. Table 10.3 provides an overview of the characteristics essential for family health and the kinds of strengths that need to exist if a family is to function effectively.

TABLE 10.3 Characteristics of a Healthy Family

Traits of a Healthy Family (Curran, 1983)
Communicates and listens
Affirms and supports one another
Teaches respect for others
Develops a sense of trust
Has a sense of play and humor
Exhibits a sense of shared responsibility
Teaches a sense of right and wrong
Has a strong sense of family in which rituals and traditions abound
Has a balance of interaction among members
Has a shared religious core
Respects the privacy of one another
Values service to others
Fosters family table time and conversation
Shares leisure time
Admits to and seeks help for problems

Family Strengths (Stinnett & DeFrain, 1985)
Commitment to family
Open communication
Showing of appreciation
Spending time together
Ability to deal with stress, conflict, and crisis

Healthy Family Characteristics (Lewis, Beavers, Gossett, & Phillips, 1976)
Patterns of problem solving
Communication style
Ability to discuss feelings
Allocation of power / negotiation
Quality of the parental relationship
Family closeness
Intimacy and autonomy
Shared values
Being tolerant of change

Healthy Family Functions (Barnhill, 1979)
Individuation
Mutuality
Flexibility
Stability
Clear perceptions
Clear role expectations
Role reciprocity
Clear generational boundaries

Even the healthiest of families is at risk for a number of stressful life events. A review of the major issues confronting families was identified by Ronald Daly, National Director for Human Development and Family Relations (as cited in Comeau, 1989). He compiled the priorities and themes being addressed by government agencies, public and private funding organizations, and public and private family social policy groups. The identified issues impacting family life and well-being are specified in Table 10.4.

Table 10.4 Issues Having an Impact on Family Life and Well–Being

Aging of the population
Teenage parenting
Child abuse and neglect
Health care costs
AIDS
Single parenting
Substance abuse
Shortage of resources to address problems of children and youth
Stress and time management
Youth suicide
Stepparenting

Other family stressors addressed by Curran (1985) and Cooper (1981) were divorce, death of a parent, frequent family relocation, insufficient family guidance, frequent absences of parent, drug and alcohol abuse, step-parenting, poor relationships between family members, mental illness, economic deprivation, and faulty communication patterns. In addition to these concerns, families also seek assistance from community mental health agencies when they encounter severe, chronic illness of a family member, violence in the family, intense anger and lack of impulse control, relocation stress, school problems and pressures, career or job problems, self-esteem issues, and difficulty with the parenting role (Copel, 1994).

It is evident that the concept of family is a complex, multifaceted one. As nurse educators strive to help students learn about and apply principles of family dynamics in their practice, they need to call upon a variety of strategies. The use of the arts and humanities, in all their richness, uniqueness, dynamism, and complexity, can aid educators in this process.

THE ARTS AND HUMANITIES IN RELATION
TO FAMILY DYNAMICS

To promote an understanding of some of the concepts contributing to the knowledge of family dynamics or to view the intricacies of the stages of the family life cycle, it is helpful to examine a variety of art forms. From literary works to great works of sculpture from past civilizations, the influence of family has been illustrated over the centuries, and these works can be used in nursing education.

Literature

Novels

To acquire comprehensive and longitudinal data on life-cycle events in families, literary works such as novels are an excellent resource. They provide data to take a student beyond the standard textbook definitions of family theory concepts, and facilitate the understanding of these concepts within the framework of a specific family situation. Use of a fictional family allows the learner to be able to amass volumes of data and perform a family assessment quickly and efficiently. Additionally, the use of a novel about a family can facilitate learning how to formulate interventions germane to family problems. By using literary examples, a learner can bypass the lengthy assessment process and go directly to using a particular theoretical model to evaluate family functioning. Table 10.5 illustrates adult literature that explores the life cycle stages and depicts many of the tasks associated with each phase.

TABLE 10.5 Examples of Novels Addressing the Life Cycle Stages

Life Cycle Stages	Literary Works
Marriage	*A Marriage Made at Woodstock* (Pelletier, 1994)
Early childbearing family	*The Pearl* (Steinbeck, 1945)
Family with preschool children	*The Child in Time* (McEwan, 1987)
Family with school-aged children	*World's Fair* (Doctorow, 1992)
Family with teenagers	*The Chosen* (Potok, 1967)
Launching family	*The Family Heart* (Dew, 1994)
Middle-aged family	*The Accidental Tourist* (Tyler, 1985)
Aging family	*On Golden Pond* (Thompson,1979)

Specific examples of fictional family life which illustrate how a family lives, experiences transitions, handles crises, and demonstrates levels of functioning over a large period of time will be briefly discussed. The novel *Family Pictures* (Miller, 1990) explores the joys and sorrows of an American family from New England struggling with the complexities of a dysfunctional marriage, the challenges of childrearing, and the chronic mental illness of a child. This novel encourages assessment and analysis of the developmental stages and family tasks that emerge throughout the family life cycle.

The book *Children's Children* (Mosco, 1981) describes the conflict around a daughter's breaking of tradition by marrying a non-Jewish man and how the family struggles and fights against the change. The impact on and the involvement of three generations is portrayed in this story through vivid escapades of family members who are in opposition to social mores and against family and religious traditions. Reading this book will not only allow one to study family dynamics and dysfunctional behaviors, but it will also provide a perspective on Jewish culture.

The saga of a southern American family who endured a chaotic and violent history struggling against the demons of the past is seen in Conroy's (1986) work, *Prince of Tides*. Each character's immeasurable suffering is depicted in addition to the ineffective coping strategies employed by each family member to handle the pain.

Anonymity: The Secret Life of an American Family (Bergman, 1995) is a book that focuses on the impact that the father's double life had on the family. It describes how the father's homosexual love affairs and subsequent death from AIDS disrupted family functioning and influenced the lives of his wife and each of the four children. The conflict between pursuing the dream of attaining economic security contrasted with the adventures of a hidden life of sexual promiscuity is the theme of the story.

Short Stories and Children's Stories

To teach children about family issues or to assist them to understand the problems and challenges that families face, educators can turn to children's literature. Table 10.6 lists a selection of children's literature that addresses some of the stressors that occur in families.

TABLE 10.6 Examples of Family Stressors Found in Children's Literature

Family Stressors	Examples in Children's Literature
Divorce	*Talk About a Family* (Greenfield, 1978)
Death of a parent	*Father Figure* (Peck, 1978)
Frequent family relocation	*Hotel Boy* (Kaufman & Kaufman, 1987)
Insufficient family guidance	*I Wish Daddy Wouldn't Drink so Much* (Vigna, 1988)
Frequent absences of parent	*Rosie and the Dance of the Dinosaurs* (Wright, 1989)
Drug and alcohol abuse	*The Edge of Next Year* (Stolz, 1974)
Stepparenting	*The Empty Chair* (Kaplan, 1978)
Poor relationships between family members	*The Quarreling Book* (Zolotow, 1963)
Mental illness	*Hummer* (Gruenberg, 1990)
Economic deprivation	*The Black Snowman* (Mendez, 1989)
Faulty communication patterns	*Where in the World Is the Perfect Family?* (Hest, 1989)
Chronic illness of a family member	*Finding a Way* (Rosenberg, 1988)
Violence in the family	*Night Riding* (Martin, 1989)
Intense anger and lack of impulse control	*I Was so Mad* (Erickson & Roffey, 1987)
Relocation stress	*Maggie Doesn't Want to Move* (O'Donnell, 1987)
School problems	*Thin Air* (Getz, 1990)
Career or job problems	*Tight Times* (Hazen, 1979)
Self-esteem issues	*The Lump in the Middle* (Adler, 1989)

Poetry

A literary form that captures the intricacies of relationships is the poem. For years poetry has been used as a medium to discuss developmental stages in families. Some examples of poems that address components of the family life cycle include "Growing Up" by U. A. Fanthorpe (1993), "The Miracle" by Maureen Hawkins (1993), "Dad" by Elaine Feinstein (1993), "Love" by Nilene Foxworth (1993), "To My Unborn Son" by Cyril Morton Thorne (1936), "We Have Lived and Loved Together" by Charles Jeffreys (1936), and "The Little Boy and the Old Man" by Shel Silverstein

(1981). Concepts of family health can be examined by reading "My Papa's Waltz" by Theodore Roethke (1975), "Any Wife or Husband" by Carol Haynes (1936), "Love" by Roy Croft (1936), and "Nobody Knows But Mother" by Mary Morrison (1936). Often attempts to explain the ironies of family life are illustrated in poems such as "Life's Scars" by Ella Wilcox (1936), "Making a Man" by Nixon Waterman (1936), "Grandmother's Old Armchair" (Anonymous, 1936), and "Where Are We Now?" by Rod McKuen (1967).

Film and Television

Many times the concepts identified from the theories on family become more vibrant and understandable when portrayed from a storyteller's perspective. Audiovisual examples of family dynamics appeal to two senses and may reinforce or give a person additional awareness and insight about family functioning that might otherwise be overlooked. Another use of literary and audiovisual examples of family life is group discussion and the application of different theoretical frameworks that can be performed based on a specific data set or case study. By providing consistency in the data base, class assignments and discussions can be better focused on certain aspects of family functioning. Most important of all, learners are attracted to and stimulated by learning opportunities that they perceive to be creative and meaningful. Each person can relate in some way to various aspects of the people or characters in these stories. Some of the various types of families exemplified in the audiovisual media are found in Table 10.7. These examples of family forms expand the traditional definition of the family.

TABLE 10.7 Examples of Family Types Found in the Audiovisual Media

Family Types	Audiovisual Media Examples
Nuclear family	*Ordinary People* (1980)
Extended family	*Joy Luck Club* (1993)
Single-parent family	*Kramer Versus Kramer* (1979)
Blended or stepfamily	*Cold Sassy Tree* (1989)
Foster family	*Free Willy* (1993)
Communal family	*Fried Green Tomatoes* (1991)

Fine Arts

Music

Another medium for enhancing one's understanding of family can be found in the lyrics of songs. Historically, family relationships have been sung about in ballads, folk songs, and the songs of popular singers. Listening to a song allows one to focus not only on the words, but also on the mood and feelings the story conveys. Music often is able to enhance both cognitive and affective learning. Table 10.8 lists some songs that focus on family needs, characteristics of both healthy and unhealthy families, painful issues that families face, and struggles within the context of relationships between family members.

Table 10.8 Examples of Songs Addressing Family Issues

Song Title and Artist	Family Issue or Concept
"Hard Headed Woman" by Cat Stevens	Traits of a healthy relationship
"Wild World" by Cat Stevens	Loss of a relationship
"Sad Lisa" by Cat Stevens	Chronic illness (schizophrenia)
"Father and Son" by Cat Stevens	Parental communication
"Allentown" by Billy Joel	Multigenerational communication
"The Night Is Still Young" by Billy Joel	Couple relationship
"Just the Way You Are" by Billy Joel	Relationship affirmation
"Operator (That's Not the Way It Feels)" by Jim Croce	Emotional cutoff
"It Doesn't Have to be that Way" by Jim Croce	Relationship loss and related depression
"Lover's Cross" by Jim Croce	Relationship conflict
"Photographs and Memories" by Jim Croce	Characteristics in healthy and unhealthy relationships
"A Time for Letting Go" by Michael Bolton	Abuse
"I'll Never Find Another You" by the Seekers	Relationship commitment
"That's the Way I've Always Heard It Should Be" by Carly Simon	Comparison of parental generation with children's generation
"Haven't Got Time for the Pain" by Carly Simon	Abuse

Song Title and Artist	Family Issue or Concept
"Cat's in the Cradle" by Harry Chapin	Repetition of family patterns
"Suspicion" by Terry Stafford	Trust in relationships
"The Great Pretender" by The Platters	Chronic illness (depression)
"Love Her Madly" by The Doors	Dysfunctional relationship
"Nowhere Man" by The Beatles	Chronic illness (general mental illness)
"Sometimes When We Touch" by Dan Hill	Communication of feelings

Painting

For centuries artists have captured the transitions, crises, and daily activities of families. By viewing a painting, a learner can visually see the artist's depiction of family transitions, crises, and quiet moments of daily living. The works of art in Table 10.9 are some examples of the profound situations that families enter. In addition to the specific works suggested, faculty may find other useful examples in *An American Vision: Three Generations of Wyeth Art* (Duff, Wyeth & Wyeth, 1987), *Norman Rockwell's America* (Finch, 1975), *Mary Cassatt: The Color Prints* (Mathews & Shapiro, 1989), *I Tell My Heart: The Art of Horace Pippin* (Stein, 1993), and *Art Past, Art Present* (Wilkins, Schultz, & Linduff, 1994); each of these collections depicts numerous family situations and could be used in studying the concept of family dynamics.

Table 10.9 Works of Art Depicting Family Situations

Family Transitions	
Jan van Eyck	"The Arnolfini Wedding Portrait"
Harmensz van Rijn Rembrandt	"The Jewish Bride"
N. C. Wyeth	"On the October Trail (A Navajo Family)"
Norman Rockwell	"Breaking Home Ties"
Norman Rockwell	"Freedom From Want"
Marc Chagall	"Lovers with Flowers"
Jan Steen	"Dancing Couple"
Leslie Emery	"This Is My Love"

Family Crises

Harmensz van Rijn Rembrandt	"Return of the Prodigal Son"
Norman Rockwell	"Easter Morning"
Norman Rockwell	"Maternity Waiting Room"
Norman Rockwell	"The Tattooist"
John De Grazia	"Navajo Wagon"
Pablo Picasso	"The Rape of the Sabine Women after David"
Pablo Picasso	"The Tragedy"
Andrew N. Wyeth	"Christina's World"

Daily Family Living

Louis LeNain	"Family of Peasants in an Interior"
Harmensz van Rijn Rembrandt	"Two Women Teaching a Child to Walk"
Angelica Kauffmann	"Cornelia, Mother of the Gracchi"
Mary S. Cassatt	"The Boating Party"
Faith Ringgold	"Tar Beach"
Horace Pippin	"Saturday Night Bath"
Mary S. Cassatt	"Maternal Caress"
Grant Wood	"American Gothic"

Sculpture

The Egyptian sculpture, "King Menkure and his Queen," which adorns the temple and entry way to the king's pyramid, is impressive and demonstrates the value of the union and positive characteristics embodied in the act of joining together as a couple. The Bernini sculpture, "Apollo and Daphne," depicts the pursuit of Daphne by Apollo and the transformation of Daphne into a tree as Apollo continues to make unwanted sexual advances. The sculpture seems to symbolize the conflict between the natural inclinations to seek out sexual gratification and the struggle of the conscious to understand and abide by the limitations of the social order. Perhaps the conflict represented by the sculpture lends itself to pondering how traits of a healthy couple or family are as challenged today as they were in ancient civilizations (Wilkins, Schultz, & Linduff, 1994).

Ancient sculpture from the Roman era such as "Reclining Couple" and "Husband and Wife" are examples of the reverence for the family (Wilkins, Schultz, & Linduff, 1994). Michelangelo's famous sculpture, "The Pietà," graphically demonstrates the suffering and pain of a mother whose son has died. An example of 19th century sculpture encompassing the concept of family is the piece "Forever Free" by Edmonia Lewis. The sculptress captures the experience of freedom for a slave couple. "The Kiss," a 20th century modern sculpture by Constantin Brancusi, depicts the tenderness of a couple's embrace (Wilkins, Schultz, & Linduff, 1994).

CONCLUSION

All of the above examples of family functioning are fraught with much conflict and pain. In looking at family frameworks the learner soon realizes that some form of conflict is inevitable. How a family chooses to respond to its problematic issues is a true test of the members' commitments to each other. The themes of being challenged, overcoming adversity, and displaying resilience and endurance characterize most families. Since the beginning of the human race, families from all cultures have used stories to teach, shape future generations, and maintain a sense of responsibility, dreams and human obligations. As educators it is important to pay attention to the use of stories in whatever form they may appear: film, sculpture, music, drama, novels, or poems. Perhaps today, more than ever, it is essential to heed the words from a fable, *Crow and Weasel*, by Barry Lopez.[1]

"I would ask you to remember only this one thing," said Badger. "The stories people tell have a way of taking care of them. If stories come to you, care for them. And learn to give them away where they are needed. Sometimes a person needs a story more than food to stay alive. That is why we put these stories in each other's memory. This is how people care for themselves."

REFERENCES

Aburdene, P., & Naisbitt, J. (1992). *Megatrends for women*. New York: Villard Books.
Adler, C. S. (1989). *The lump in the middle*. Boston: Clarion Books.

1. From Lopez, B. (1990). *Crow and weasel* (p. 48). San Francisco: North Point Press. Used by permission.

Anonymous. (1936). "Grandmother's old arm chair." In H. Felleman, *The best loved poems of the American people* (p. 288). New York: Doubleday.

Aponte, H. J., & Van Deusen, J. M. (1981). Structural family therapy. In A. S. Gurman & D. P. Kniskern (Eds.), *Handbook of family therapy* (pp. 310–360). New York: Brunner/Mazel.

Barnhill, L. (1979). Healthy family systems. *Family Coordinator, 29,* 94–100.

Bergman, S. (1995). *Anonymity: The secret life of an American family.* New York: Warner Books.

Bowen, M. (1978). *Family therapy in clinical practice.* New York: Jason Aronson.

Carter, E., & McGoldrick, M. (1980). The family life cycle and family therapy: An overview. In E. Carter & M. McGoldrick (Eds.), *The family life cycle: A framework for family therapy* (pp. 3–28). New York: Gardner Press.

Comeau, J. (1989). Issues impacting family life and well being. *Family Information Services, 3,* 5–10.

Conroy, P. (1986). *Prince of tides.* New York: Bantam Books.

Cooper, C. L. (1981). *The stress check: Coping with the stressors of life and work.* Englewood Cliffs, NJ: Prentice–Hall.

Copel, L. C. (1994). [Issues families bring to community mental health centers]. Unpublished raw data.

Croft, R. (1936). "Love." In H. Felleman (Selected by), *The best loved poems of the American people* (p. 25). Garden City, NY: Doubleday & Co.

Curran, D. (1983). *Traits of a healthy family.* New York: Ballantine.

Curran, D. (1985). *Stress and the healthy family.* Minneapolis, MN: Winston Press.

Dew, R. F. (1994). *The family heart: A memoir of when our son came out.* New York: Addison Wesley.

Doctorow, E. L. (1992). *World's fair.* New York: Random House.

Duff, J. H., Wyeth, A., & Wyeth, J. (1987). *An American vision: Three generations of Wyeth art.* Boston: Little, Brown and Company.

Duvall, E. (1977). *Marriage and family development* (5th ed.). Philadelphia: Lippincott.

Erickson, K., & Roffey, M. (1987). *I was so mad.* New York: Viking Penguin.

Fanthorpe, V. A. (1993). "Growing up." In I. Linthwaite (Ed.), *Ain't I a woman! A book of womens poetry from around the world* (p. 6). New York: Wings Books.

Fawcett, J. (1977). The relationship between identification and patterns of change in spouses' body images during and after pregnancy. *International Nursing Review, 14,* 199–213.

Feinstein, E. (1993). "Dad." In I. Linthwaite (Ed.), *Ain't I a woman! A book of womens poetry from around the world* (p. 100). New York: Wings Books.

Finch, C. (1975). *Norman Rockwell's America*. New York: Harry N. Abrams, Inc.

Foxworth, N. O. (1993). "Love." In I. Linthwaite (Ed.), *Ain't I a woman! A book of womens poetry from around the world* (p. 174). New York: Wings Books.

Getz, D. (1990). *Thin air*. New York: Harper Collins.

Gillis, C. L., Highley, B. L., Roberts, B. M., & Martinson, I. M. (1989). *Toward a science of family nursing*. Menlo Park, CA: Addison–Wesley.

Greenfield, E. (1978). *Talk about a family*. Philadelphia: Lippincott.

Gruenberg, L. (1990). *Hummer*. New York: Houghton Mifflin.

Hawkins, M. (1993). "The miracle." In I. Linthwaite (Ed.), *Ain't I a woman! A book of women's poetry from around the world* (p. 77). New York: Wings Books.

Haynes, C. (1936). "Any wife or husband." In H. Felleman (selected by), *The best loved poems of the American people* (p. 23). Garden City, NY: Doubleday & Co.

Hazen, B.S. (1979). *Tight times*. Viking Press.

Hest, A. (1989). *Where in the world is the perfect family?* New York: Clarion Books.

Hill, R., & Rodgers, R. H. (1964). The developmental approach. In H. T. Christensen (Ed.), *Handbook of marriage and the family* (pp. 171–211). Chicago: Rand McNally.

Holaday, B. (1981). Maternal response to their chronically ill infants' attachment behavior of crying. *Nursing Research, 30,* 343–348.

Janosik, E., & Green, E. (1992). *Family life: Process and practice*. Boston: Jones and Bartlett.

Jeffreys, C. (1936). "We have lived and loved together." In H. Felleman (selected by), *The best loved poems of the American people* (p. 34). Garden City, NY: Doubleday & Co.

Kaplan, B. (1978). *The empty chair*. New York: Harper & Row.

Kaufman, C., & Kaufman, G. (1987). *Hotel boy*. New York: Atheneum Publishers.

Knafl, K. A., & Deatrick, J. A. (1987). Conceptualizing family response to a child's chronic illness or disability. *Family Relations, 36,* 300–304.

Lewis, J. M., Beavers, W. R., Gossett, J. T., & Phillips, V. A. (1976). *No single thread: Psychological health in family systems*. New York: Brunner/Mazel.

Lopez, B. (1990). *Crow and weasel*. San Francisco: North Point Press.

Martin, K. (1989). *Night riding*. New York: Knopf.

Mathews, N. M., & Shapiro, B. S. (1989). *Mary Cassatt: The color prints*. New York: Harry N. Abrams, Inc.

May, R. (1972). *Psychology and the human dilemma*. Princeton, NJ: D. Van Nostrand.

McEwan, I. (1987). *The child in time*. Boston: Houghton Mifflin.

McKuen. R. (1967). Where are we now? In R. McKuen, *Lonesome cities* (p. 93). New York: Random House.

Mendez, P. (1989). *The black snowman*. New York: Scholastic Inc.

Miller, S. (1990). *Family pictures*. New York: Harper & Row.

Minuchin, S., Montalvo, B., Guerney, J., Rosman, B., & Schumer, F. (1967). *Families of the slums*. New York: Basic Books.

Minuchin, S., Rosman, B. L., & Baker, L. (1978). *Psychosomatic families*. Cambridge, MA: Harvard University Press.

Morrison, M. (1936). "Nobody knows but mother." In H. Felleman, *The best loved poems of the American people* (p. 381). New York: Doubleday.

Mosco, M. (1981). *Children's children*. New York: Harper & Row.

O'Donnell, E. L. (1987). *Maggie doesn't want to move*. New York: Four Winds Press.

Olson, D. H., Sprenkle, D. H., & Russell, C. S. (1979). Circumplex model of marital and family systems, I: Cohesion and adaptability dimensions, family types, and clinical applications. *Family Process, 18,* 3–28.

Peck, R. (1978). *Father figure*. New York: Viking Press.

Pelletier, C. (1994). *A marriage made at Woodstock*. New York: Crown.

Potok, C. (1967). *The chosen*. New York: Fawcett Crest.

Roethke, T. (1975). "My Papa's waltz." In T. Roethke, *The collected poems of Theodore Roethke* (p. 43). New York: Anchor Books.

Rosenberg, M. (1988). *Finding a way: Living with exceptional brothers and sisters*. New York: Lothrop, Lee, and Shephard Books.

Rowe, G. P. (1966). The developmental conceptual framework to the study of the family. In F. I. Nye, & F. M. Berardo (Eds.), *Emerging conceptual frameworks in family analysis* (pp. 198–223). New York: Macmillan.

Satir, V. (1972). *Peoplemaking*. Palo Alto, CA: Science and Behavior Books.

Satir, V. (1982). The therapist and family therapy: Process model. In A. M. Horne & M. M. Ohlsen (Eds.), *Family counseling and therapy* (pp. 14–32). Itasca, IL: F.E. Peacock.

Satir, V., Stachwiak, J., & Taschmen, H. (1977). *Helping families to change*. New York: Jason Aronson.

Silverstein, S. (1981). "The little boy and the old man." In S. Silverstein, *A light in the attic* (p. 95). New York: Harper & Row.

Smith, L. (1983). A conceptual model of families incorporating an adolescent mother and child into the household. *Advances in Nursing Science, 6,* 45–60.

Stanton, M. D., & Todd, T. C. (1979). Structural family therapy with drug addicts. In E. Kaufman & P. Kaufman (Eds.), *The family therapy of drug and alcohol abuse* (pp. 55–70). New York: Gardner Press.

Stein, J. E. (1993). *I tell my heart: The art of Horace Pippin.* New York: Universe Publishing.

Steinbeck, J. (1945). *The pearl.* New York: Viking Press.

Stinnett, N., & DeFrain, J. (1985). *Secrets of strong families.* Boston: Little, Brown.

Stolz, M. (1974). *The edge of next year.* New York: Harper & Row.

Thorne, C. M. (1936). "To my unborn son." In H. Felleman (selected by), *The best loved poems of the American people* (p. 24). Garden City, NY: Doubleday & Co.

Toman, W. (1969). *Family constellation.* New York: Springer Publishing Co.

Thompson, E. (1979). *On golden pond.* New York: Dodd, Mead.

Tyler, A. (1985). *The accidental tourist.* New York: Knopf.

Vigna, J. (1988). *I wish daddy didn't drink so much.* Morton Grove, IL: Whitman & Company.

Walsh, F. (1993). Conceptualizations of normal family processes. In F. Walsh (Ed.), *Normal family processes* (2nd ed., pp. 1–28). New York: Guilford Press.

Waterman, N. (1936). "Making a Man." In H. Felleman (selected by), *The best loved poems of the American people* (p. 413). Garden City, NY: Doubleday & Co.

Watzlawick, P., Beavin, J., & Jackson, D. (1967). *Pragmatics of human communication.* New York: Norton.

Weakland, J. (1976). Communication theory and clinical change. In P. Guerin (Ed.), *Family therapy and practice* (pp. 111–128). New York: Gardner Press.

Wilcox, E. (1936). "Life's scars." In H. Felleman (selected by), *The best loved poems of the American people* (p. 645). Garden City, NY: Doubleday & Co.

Wilkins, D. G., Schultz, B., & Linduff, K. M. (1994). *Art past, art present* (2nd ed.). New York: Harry N. Abrams, Inc.

Wright, B. R. (1989). *Rosie and the dance of the dinosaurs.* New York: Holiday House.

Wynne, L. (1978). *Beyond the doublebind.* New York: Brunner/Mazel.

Zolotow, C. (1963). *The quarreling book.* New York: Harper & Row.

11

Health and Illness

Catherine Todd Magel, EdD, RN

All nursing care focuses on health. Although there are many nursing roles, each role can be related to the promotion of health of an individual, group, or community. It would seem that consensus about the characterization of health must, therefore, exist; but the literature provides a variety of definitions and models pertaining to health. Initially these competing views may be overwhelming, but the diversity can actually be helpful to nursing practice. One's view of health is relative to past and present experiences. The greater a nurse's exposure to multiple views of health, the more likely an appreciation of a client's unique view of health can be gained. This discussion focuses on multiple views of health and includes overviews of various models which characterize health. Concepts relating to illness also are addressed, and varying views which characterize illness are provided.

HEALTH

An individual's characterization of health is reflective of past and present experiences; physical, psychological, and social attributes; and cultural and spiritual influences. This personal characterization can change over time due to the influence of aging, illness, and exposure to new ideas and experiences. Since each individual's characterization of health is unique, the nurse's and patient's goals related to health may differ greatly. The nurse must gain insight into the patient's values about health to provide patient-centered nursing care.

A simple description of health is that it is the state which exists in the absence of illness, but this is an inadequate and, in some instances, an inaccurate statement. This description implies that health and illness are either-or states, and it offers no recognition of the multiple factors which make health a dynamic state that changes according to internal and external influences. Rather than struggling to identify a single definition of health that is universally accepted, a review of various factors which can influence an individual's perception of health appears to be more informative. While the presence and dominance of particular factors will vary among individuals, the nurse can gain an appreciation of the client's perception of health by considering these factors.

FACTORS INFLUENCING PERCEPTIONS OF HEALTH

If health is viewed as a dynamic state which is personally defined, then it is necessary to describe the factors which play a role in defining, influencing, and changing an individual's perception of health. These factors may be categorized as intrinsic factors and extrinsic factors.

Intrinsic Factors

Genetic Component

The genetic endowment of an individual can create limitations in mental or physical functioning and increase risks for particular pathologies. Each of these can affect the perceptions of health of the individual.

Intellectual Dimension

The cognitive ability of an individual can influence perceptions of health as well as knowledge about attaining or maintaining health.

Psychological Variables

Perceptions and misconceptions of reality, as well as personality, emotions, and mood, all can affect an individual's view of health. Because each of these variables may change over time or be influenced by the situation, the view of health can be expected to change as well.

Spiritual Influences

One's beliefs about the meaning and purpose of life, sources of happiness, and the role of spirituality can affect feelings of control of one's health, as well as acceptable actions to attain or maintain health.

Physiological Variables

The biological functioning or malfunctioning of body parts and the integration of biological functioning into socially acceptable patterns influences the individual's perceptions of health.

Extrinsic Factors

Economic Variables

The financial capabilities which provide for shelter, food, health care, leisure activities and the purchase of goods and services affects perceptions of health.

Social Factors

The roles of the individual, availability of others for physical assistance and emotional support, and the place of an individual within a given society impacts on health perceptions.

Cultural Factors

The identification with the cultural beliefs and values of a particular group influences perceptions of health and acceptable behaviors regarding health.

Environmental Factors

The geographical location of an individual determines the availability of some resources, and the quality of things such as water and air. All of these factors impose limitations which can affect perceptions of health.

HEALTH MODELS

The use of a model to present concepts and ideas pertinent to health can be a way to gain insight into the components influencing an individual's view of health. The benefit of a model is that it shows relationships between parts and thereby provides a framework for application to practice. Several models are presented here to show the diversity which exists in health models and to increase the likelihood that one may be appropriate in a particular situation.

Health–Illness Continuum Model

The Health–Illness Continuum Model provides a representation of health in terms of a scale or continuum, with high-level health being at one end and severe illness or death at the opposite end (Neuman, 1990). A wide range of varying states of health, thus, is possible, and there is recognition that many variables can influence an individual's place along the continuum.

The health–illness continuum provides a way for patients to indicate their personal current health status. This information can be quite revealing, as physical and psychosocial conditions can influence the patient's perceptions but may not be obvious to the nurse who is obtaining assessment data. A limitation of the Health–Illness Continuum Model is that determining a point between two extremes, which represents one's current health status, is difficult since it is subjective, imprecise, and influenced by many factors, as noted.

High-Level Wellness Model

Described and later modified by Dunn (1959; 1977), the High-Level Wellness Model is directed toward helping patients achieve their fullest health potential. The patient is viewed as maintaining both balance and purposeful direction in the environment, with the integration of health practices occurring at increasing levels throughout life.

This can be applied to individuals, families, and groups. In addition, health promotion and illness-prevention activities—rather than interventions to treat illness—are the focus. The goal of high-level wellness is optimum functioning through integration of multiple approaches to promote health. High-level wellness is viewed as a dynamic state requiring ongoing attention. The High-Level Wellness Model's use presumes acceptance of the goal of maximizing the health potential, which may not be the priority in a particular situation.

Health Promotion Model

The Health Promotion Model was designed by Pender (1987) and is directed at increasing an individual's well-being. It focuses on the personal aspects which influence an individual's participation in health-promoting behaviors. Because the model's emphasis is on the individual, it is not appropriate for use with families or groups.

The Health Promotion Model provides a list of potential factors to consider in assessing the patient, thus increasing the consistency and reliability of the assessments. The modifying factors may change over time, so considering these provides information about the current potential for health-promoting behavior by the patient, and permits individual differences related to time and situation.

ILLNESS

As with health, an individual's past and present experiences; physical, psychological, and social attributes; and cultural and spiritual dimensions all influence his or her characterization of illness. One's perception of illness greatly affects the activities in which one engages, the help one seeks or accepts, and the roles one enacts. The characterization of illness can change over time due to developmental level, experiences, aging, and exposure to new ideas. Situational factors also can influence one's perception of illness, and the importance or urgency of other commitments may impact on whether or not one labels oneself sick.

Illness may be examined in terms of contributing or causative factors, the experience of being ill, and the time factors involved in illness and recovery. In each instance, personal perceptions influence beliefs, expectations, and behaviors. In order to be effective in providing patient-centered care, the nurse must gain insight into the patient's perceptions about illness, correct misconceptions, and accept those aspects which have contributed to the patient's beliefs. Information about various conceptions pertaining to illness, and factors influencing perceptions of illness can enrich nurses' assessments and their appreciation of patients' beliefs.

CHARACTERISTICS OF ILLNESS

Illness may be described as the opposite of health, but such a description presents an either-or situation and ignores the range which may exist between the two experiences. Illness is a personally defined state, relative to the same factors which affect perceptions of health; thus it is necessary to explore the factors that influence illness, if one wants to characterize the concept.

Open Systems

If one views the human being as an open system in continuous interaction with the environment, illness may be seen as causing a change in the system so that it no longer forms a unified functioning whole. The interrelatedness of the parts of the system supports the idea of the mind and the body existing in an interdependent relationship, and it enables understanding of how mental illness can affect physical functioning and vice-versa.

Homeostasis

The principle of homeostasis also is pertinent to a discussion about open systems and illness. Homeostasis is the process of maintaining stability in an open system by continuous response to stimuli. Therefore, homeostasis is a dynamic, rather than static, state. Illness may be viewed as a disruption to which the system responds in an effort to reestablish homeostasis. Because the process of reestablishing homeostasis requires energy in various forms, the availability of resources will influence the time needed and the ability of the system to respond to the illness and move toward homeostasis. In some situations, there is a quick recovery; in others, a prolonged but successful process occurs. Finally, in situations in which depletion of resources occurs before homeostasis can be reestablished, the outcome can be exhaustion and ongoing illness, or death.

Stress

The work of Hans Selye (1976) in describing stress and the complex human responses to stress relates to the previous discussion about open systems and homeostasis and adds further insight into the dimensions of illness. Stressors may be physical or emotional, internal or external to the body, and require the body to respond in some way. However, the response by the body is not specific; both

positive and negative emotions elicit similar biophysical responses. Stress permeates life, and the body's ongoing ability to make
adjustments in response to stress determines whether or not one
becomes ill and whether or not one survives illness.

FACTORS INFLUENCING PERCEPTIONS OF ILLNESS

Many factors affect perceptions of illness, and a number of these
factors were presented as ones that also influence perceptions of
health. The factors were categorized as intrinsic and extrinsic and
include: genetic components, intellectual dimension, psychological
variables, spiritual influences, physiological variables, economic
variables, social factors, cultural factors, and the physical environment. Additionally, there are several factors that may be identified
as pertinent to how one perceives illness.

Duration of Illness

The length of time one expects to be ill affects the response to being
labeled as such. How realistic one's time frame is depends on the
accuracy of information received about the nature and usual
course of a particular illness, knowledge of others with similar illnesses, and one's past experiences when ill. Because some individuals use time estimations of illness to determine how long they
will continue with therapies and when certain activities can be
resumed, the accuracy of these time estimations greatly influences
the completion of desired plans of intervention.

Acute and Chronic Illness

An acute illness often occurs without warning, thus one has no
way to prepare physically or emotionally. When one is surprised,
disbelief often results and the patient who unexpectedly becomes
acutely ill may not be able to comprehend information or instructions during the initial period of the illness. Nursing care focuses
on supporting the patient during this time and also supporting the
family and friends who are in contact with the patient. Although
the patient's significant others also may be in a state of disbelief,
their physical health places them at an advantage in coping, and

they often are needed to guide the patient in decision making about plans and therapies.

A chronic illness creates limitations in the individual which persist. Thus, chronic illnesses require changes in lifestyle to accommodate interventions and limitations imposed by the illness. How well the individual can integrate these changes depends on a number of factors including acceptance of the illness, motivation to comply with suggested regimens, and benefits perceived from the compliance. Because of the sustained nature and duration of chronic illnesses, families and friends often find that the individual's illness has an impact on their lives, with a variety of potential responses and outcomes apparent. A chronic illness can affect every aspect of life; therefore, decisions about diet, transportation, medication administration, therapies, household chores, and living arrangements all may be necessary.

Seriousness of Illness

Whether or not one believes an illness to be serious will also influence how one perceives the illness. Knowledge about the nature of the illness can be gained through information offered by professionals or the media, from individuals who have experienced the illness, or from secondhand reports of those who have known such individuals. Therefore, accuracy can be affected through misinformation or misunderstanding of correct information. If a patient is unable to accept the fact that a serious illness exists, interventions to restore and promote health may be complicated by what the patient perceives.

Family and friends are likely to experience changes in the relationship with someone diagnosed with a serious illness. While expected to serve as a support to the patient, these others may be examining issues in their own lives and may actually withdraw from the patient as they focus on their own emotional responses and their own mortality. It is during this time that nurses need to consider the patient and the significant others as each needs acceptance and support when the threat of serious illness becomes a reality.

Meaning of Illness

How illness affects an individual depends on a number of factors including the meaning of the illness for the individual at that particular time. The meaning of illness is probably the most personal aspect of illness for anyone and often not part of the conscious awareness. Cultural and spiritual experiences greatly affect the meanings associated with illness, and the variety of possibilities makes prediction of anyone's response difficult, if not impossible. What is important in providing nursing care is realizing that a wide variety of interpretations exists, and patient behaviors and responses may be related to these underlying beliefs.

It may be impossible to determine the meaning of an illness for an individual because part of the person's beliefs may be unconscious influences on behavior. But illness can activate the search for meaning, and clues that this is occurring are gleaned from listening to the questions a patient raises and the statements made about factors presumed to be related to the illness. The patient may withdraw while pondering the meaning of illness, and family and friends need to be made aware that it is not unusual for one to try to find meaning in one's experience.

SUMMARY

The concepts of health and illness are integral to nursing care. One's views of health and illness are influenced by personal experiences, both past and present. When providing nursing care it is necessary to gain an appreciation of the views of health and illness held by others, so that the care that is provided is truly patient centered.

THE ARTS AND HUMANITIES IN RELATION TO HEALTH AND ILLNESS

Individuals define the concepts of health and illness in unique and personal ways. In addition to understanding the various factors that affect individuals' perceptions of these dynamic concepts, nurses need to be aware of what it means to be healthy or to be ill. Thus, faculty need to identify teaching methods that help students explore the nature of these experiences, and the effects that they have on all aspects of life. Because the arts and humanities provide insight into the human condition, their use may enable students to understand health and illness from a broader perspective.

Literature

Novels

Numerous authors have described personal experiences, or those of family members, with health and illness. They have explored such disorders as heart disease, *Heart Sounds* (Lear, 1980); cystic fibrosis, *Alex: The Life of a Child* (Deford, 1983); genetic abnormalities, *Lisa H* (Severo, 1985) and *Journey* (Massie & Massie, 1976); physical disability, *The Body's Memory* (Stewart, 1989); and mental illness, *Darkness Visible* (Styron, 1990) and *Girl, Interrupted* (Kaysen, 1993). In each of these accounts, the authors shared the effects of the illness on all aspects of their lives, their interactions with the health care system, and their need to find meaning in their experience.

Bed Number Ten (Baier & Schomaker, 1986), an honest and graphic account of a woman's experience with Guillain-Barré syndrome, is an excellent resource for nursing faculty. In the book, Sue Baier details the feelings of dependency, helplessness, fear, and loneliness associated with total body paralysis. Because Sue was awake and alert throughout her ordeal, she was aware not only of the care and concern of many health care professionals, but also of the insensitivity of others: "Do they know how this feels? I am constantly alone. The nurses are close by in that nursing station, but they are busy talking . . . how can they be so indifferent and cold?" (p. 37).

This is a compelling book. The brisk, clear narrative enables the reader to "be" in Sue's situation, and thus, it provides insight into a rare human experience. Because it is difficult to avoid being affected emotionally by this story, it might be helpful to have students express their reactions to it in writing. The introspection associated with writing may enhance students' understanding of this woman's story.

Gilda Radner's (1989) account of her battle with cancer, *It's Always Something*, is both humorous and poignant. Although the popular actress succumbed to the disease, her intimate sharing of the myriad emotions associated with cancer—for example, the feeling of loss of control that cancer imposed on her—is invaluable to those who seek to understand its overwhelming impact. Through this book students can learn to help patients adjust to the uncertainty of cancer and find ways to live within the limitations that it imposes.

In the book, *A Bomb in the Brain* (Fishman, 1988), the author candidly describes his own brain surgery and subsequent diagnosis of epilepsy, and tells a personal story about the response of his family and friends to his condition, his personal feelings about the experience, and the changes it affects in his life. As such, this book truly captures the affective aspects of a condition that has long been surrounded by myth and misunderstanding. Steve Fishman's story emphasizes the need to listen to patients so that their care encompasses more than the application of technical knowledge.

The struggle of a young anorexic to control the hospital regime is depicted in the novel, *Life-Size* (Shute, 1992). Josie, a graduate school drop-out, weighs 69.5 pounds; she spends her days in the hospital deciding what to eat and what not to eat, and trying to convince herself that she is in charge. Through Josie's musings about her body's needs and her obsession with her diet, the book reveals the spiritual nature of anorexia and the courage that it takes to recover. Because students may respond to this story in a personal manner, faculty need to be sensitive to their need to express their views about Josie's experience.

Short Stories

Dancing Against the Darkness (Petrow, 1990) contains the stories of individuals who have AIDS or HIV, and describes their efforts to live with hope and dignity in the face of insurmountable odds. In preparing the stories, the author also interviewed the patients' families, friends, and colleagues. The focus on the individuals' stories humanizes this disease, and reminds the reader of the impact of AIDS on all aspects of life. This book offers students the opportunity to reflect on their own attitudes toward AIDS patients and their fears about contracting AIDS in the workplace. The stories could be used as case studies; they are a nonthreatening way for students to become acquainted with the human experience of AIDS.

Children who are ill have needs and concerns not unlike those of adult patients. This often forgotten point, and the lessons that can be learned from children as they face the challenges of illness, are emphasized in the sensitive and technically accurate book, *The Boy Who Felt No Pain* (Marion, 1990). In the short story, *Kevin's Question*, for example, a young boy learns that his condition is related to his mother's alcoholism; his initial anger gives way to understanding when the doctor explains, "she can't control her drinking any more than you can control the fact that you've got spina bifida" (p. 90). The stories in this collection provide topics for discussion such as the emotional needs of ill children, the effects of children's illnesses on their families, and ethical dilemmas encountered in pediatrics.

The Man Who Mistook His Wife for a Hat and Other Clinical Tales (Sacks, 1985) is a collection of 20 stories that detail the experiences of individuals afflicted with neurologic disorders. In the preface the author emphasizes the need to include the "patient's essential being" (p. xiv) in any discussion of a clinical history. Thus, although the disorders described in the stories are, indeed, bizarre, one comes to know the patients in terms of their uniquely human qualities and needs. These stories can help students "see" beyond diseases to the individuals who experience them.

Children' Stories

The impact of Alzheimer's disease on the children and grandchildren of its victims is described, at a very basic level, in the book, *Maria's Grandma Gets Mixed Up* (Sanford, 1989). The family learns to take care of Grandma, and accepts the fact that there is no cure. This book could be useful to students during a clinical experience in the community. As more families care for elderly individuals in their homes, nurses need to identify strategies that address the needs of all the members of the family. An awareness of how it feels to have a grandparent with Alzheimer's could enhance students' ability to help a young child deal with this difficult situation.

Although not written specifically for children, *I Will Sing Life* (Berger, Lithwick, & Seven Campers, 1992), is, in a very real sense, a children's book, because it describes children's experiences with lifethreatening illnesses in their own words. All the children who tell their stories in this book have attended Paul Newman's Hole in the Wall Gang Camp; their stories reflect their courage, spirit, and determination to survive. Again, this collection depicts the experience of illness and the deep emotions it triggers. Students can share the children's wisdom and their sense of hope with patients of all ages.

Poetry

Robert Frost (1949, pp.171–172) described the loss of a *young* boy's hand, and eventually of his life, in the graphic poem, "Out, Out." The boy's hand is amputated accidently as he works on a woodpile at his family's farm. At first he tried to deny what happened, and then he accepted the reality and thought his life was over. Finally, unable to cope with such a traumatic loss, the boy dies. This poem expresses the meaning of the loss of a body part in a brief, yet explicit, manner. It might be instructive to have students write an alternative ending to this poem that reflects their understanding of the human need to verbalize feelings about such an experience.

Two of John Stone's poems are particularly useful when teaching health and illness. In "He Makes a House Call" (1980a), a physician describes how different a patient seems in the context of his own home where he is in charge of everything, including life. The poem, "The Girl in the Hall" (1980b), expresses a physician's perspective as he returns from amputating a patient's leg; he is sensitive to the patient's loss and recognizes that he may gradually get used to his condition. Both poems emphasize the insight that health care professionals need to cultivate to address patients' needs in a holistic and humanistic manner. Perhaps students could be encouraged to write a poem that expresses their understanding of a particular patient's experience. The process of reflecting on and articulating one's feelings in writing can enhance self-knowledge and foster sensitivity.

Films and Television

In the film, *Regarding Henry* (1991), a high-powered lawyer with little time for anything but work reevaluates his life after sustaining a brain injury. During the long weeks and months of his rehabilitation, he comes to recognize the people and simple pleasures that give meaning to his life. Although the film tends to romanticize a difficult situation, it does depict the impact of Henry's long illness on his ability to work, his financial situation, and his personal relationships. This film can help students understand the importance of listening to patients as they reflect on the meaning of their experiences and try to adjust to the changes that they may have to make in their lives.

Three recent films depict the dramatic impact of paralysis on every aspect of a patient's life. In *Passion Fish* (1993), a successful young actress returns to her home in rural Louisiana after becoming paralyzed in an accident. The film is a frank portrayal of the difficulties she experiences in adjusting to her disability and in finding a nurse with whom she can communicate. By providing a brief introduction to the plot, faculty can use selected scenes from this film without diminishing its impact. One scene, in particular, in which the woman falls on the floor and lies there for hours in utter frustration and helplessness, can be appreciated outside the context of the film without much difficulty.

The director of the film, *The Waterdance* (1992), was paralyzed in an accident, and used his personal experience to provide a most authentic perspective on the depiction of his disability. In this film, a young novelist, paralyzed in a hiking accident, goes to a rehabilitation center and encounters fellow paraplegics from a variety of cultural backgrounds. The different attitudes and life experiences of the other characters enhance the effectiveness of this film.

Finally, *My Left Foot* (1990), the film autobiography of artist-writer Christy Brown, presents disability in an intense manner. Brown, crippled with cerebral palsy, is a feisty, difficult survivor who receives tremendous support and encouragement from his mother. He uses this support to become a successful artist and bring his disability to the public.

Because all three of these films are candid and realistic, they can sensitize students to the serious implications of long-term disability. In addition, they address the role of health care professionals and families in the care of severely disabled individuals.

Terms of Endearment (1983) traces the mercurial relationship between a mother and daughter from the young woman's childhood to her untimely death from cancer. The film excels in its ability to convey the impact of terminal illness on the patient's family. In one unforgettable scene, the mother, played by Shirley MacLaine, screams at the nurses that her daughter is in pain and needs her medication. It would be a truly insensitive nurse who could view this scene and not be affected by its poignant message. The film also provides students with the opportunity to reflect on such topics as end-of-life decisions and the sick role.

Magazine-type programs on television occasionally provide in-depth coverage of a health-illness issue or concern. Because of the tendency of these programs to sensationalize health care issues, faculty should warn students to keep an open mind when viewing such presentations. Students also could be instructed to critique the technical accuracy of the information that is presented.

Television has addressed AIDS using the teledrama format. The "Ryan White Story" was a moving depiction of the tragic story of a young hemophiliac who was ostracized by neighbors and friends when he contracted the disease. Although the program humanized AIDS, it did so by portraying an uncommon victim rather than a male homosexual or intravenous drug abuser. Nonetheless, the program did convey the negative treatment that sometimes is directed toward AIDS victims and the ignorance that often underlies such behavior. For this reason it could be used to help students identify their own attitudes and biases toward the disease and those who suffer from it.

Fine Arts

Drama

The 1994 play, *Night Sky*, by Susan Yankowitz, is the story of Anna, a successful astronomer, who becomes aphasic after a car accident. The play depicts Anna's struggle to communicate and her gradual acceptance of herself as a different person. Her desire to return to her work and to maintain her relationship with her daughter and her lover motivate her to succeed. Through the play one gains a very real sense of what it is like to be aphasic. In addition, students could identify the factors in Anna's current situation and the experiences from her past that affected her ability to cope with her disability.

Painting

Pain is a subjective phenomenon that is difficult for individuals to describe. Nonetheless, nurses need an understanding of pain in order to help patients cope with it. "Gripping Headache," by Raymond Dorow, is a remarkably graphic work of art that depicts a man in agonizing pain from a chronic headache. In the painting, the man's mouth is agape in agony, his eyes are wide open, and his hands are clutching the sides of his head; a hand is seen pulling what appears to be brain tissue through the top of his skull. The realistic conceptualization of pain depicted in this work moves one to an immediate sense of empathy for this man's suffering. After describing their response to this painting, students could be directed to discuss what they would do if they encountered this situation in practice: "What might you do first?", "How would you speak to this patient?", and "What would you ask him?", are examples of questions that could stimulate critical thinking about the nature of and the nurse's response to human pain.

Psychological pain is as difficult as physical pain to describe and quantify. Edvard Munch's "The Scream" is a powerful image of anxiety that engenders strong feelings in those who view the painting. It depicts the distorted figure of a man standing on a bridge with the sun setting behind him. The man is clutching the sides of his head; his mouth is drawn in an oval shape that suggests the emission of a scream. Students could be instructed to write a survey description of this man's appearance and behavior, and indicate what additional data they would need before they could generate a nursing diagnosis. It is hoped that students would recognize the need to communicate with this patient in an attempt to understand his feelings.

Photography

Epitaphs for the Living: Words and Images in the Time of AIDS (Howard, 1989) is a book of photographs of 68 people with AIDS, accompanied by statements from each of the individuals or from friends or family members. Although many of the individuals appear healthy, others seem frail, and still others are depicted in their hospital beds. The photographs are of men and women who represent a variety of cultures and who span the spectrum of lifestyles and socioeconomic levels. The emotions expressed in the statements are deeply personal and describe feelings of anger, loneliness, hope, fear, and love.

This collection offers a glimpse of people who have been afflicted with AIDS and the meaning this experience has for them. In addition, it helps to dispel stereotypes about the disease. Faculty could encourage students to respond verbally to the statements in a manner that expresses their awareness of the patient's experience.

Alan Brightman (1984) emphasizes that *Ordinary Moments: The Disabled Experience* is not about the "subject of disability" (p. 4). The book, a combination of photographs and stories, is an attempt to uncover the experience of disability and to educate society about who the disabled really are and how they want to be perceived. The collection focuses on eight individuals and includes such people as Nancy who is deaf, and Ed who has muscular dystrophy. The sensitive and honest approach of this book makes it especially useful to stimulate discussion about stereotypes regarding disability, as well as strategies that might be helpful in providing care that reflects the needs of the disabled rather than those of the nurse.

CONCLUSION

The notion of patient-centered care requires that nurses understand the complex and dynamic concepts of health and illness from a humanistic as well as a theoretical perspective. Knowledge regarding the various factors that influence health beliefs and behaviors can be obtained from textbooks and lectures. An awareness of the affective component of these concepts, however, must be achieved by listening to patients as they describe the meaning of health and illness in their lives, an awareness that can also be developed from interactions with a variety of art forms. In addition, reflection on the arts and humanities can sensitize students to the need to listen to patients, to acknowledge that patients' beliefs about health and illness affect their goals, and to plan care that is directed toward patients' unique needs and objectives.

REFERENCES

Baier, S., & Schomaker, M. (1985). *Bed number ten*. Boca Raton, FL: CRC Press, Inc.

Berger, L., Lithwick, D., & Seven Campers. (1992). *I will sing life*. New York: Little, Brown and Company.

Brightman, A. (1984). *Ordinary moments: The disabled experience*. Baltimore, MD: University Park Press.

Deford, F. (1983). *Alex: The life of a child*. Baltimore, MD: Cystic Fibrosis Foundation.

Dunn, H. (1959). High-level wellness for man and society. *American Journal of Public Health, 49*, 789–794.

Dunn, H. (1977). What high level wellness means. *Health Values, 1*, 9–16.

Fishman, S. (1988). *A bomb in the brain*. New York: Charles Scribner's Sons.

Frost, R. (1949). *Complete poems of Robert Frost*. New York: Henry Holt and Co.

Howard, B. (1989). *Epitaphs for the living: Words and images in the time of AIDS*. Dallas, TX: Southern Methodist University Press.

Kaysen, S. (1993). *Girl, interrupted*. New York: Vintage Books.

Lear, M. (1980). *Heartsounds*. New York: Pocket Books.

Marion, R. (1990). *The boy who felt no pain*. Reading, MA: Addison–Wesley.

Massie, R., & Massie, S. (1976). *Journey*. New York: Warner Books.

Neuman, B. (1990). Health as a continuum based on the Neuman systems model. *Nursing Science Quarterly, 3,* 129–135.

Pender, N. (1987). *Health promotion in nursing practice* (2nd ed.). Norwalk, CT: Appleton & Lange.

Petrow, S. (1990). *Dancing against the darkness*. Lexington, MA: D.C. Heath and Company.

Radner, G. (1989). *It's always something*. New York: Avon Books.

Sacks, O. (1985). *The man who mistook his wife for a hat and other clinical tales.* New York: Summit Books.

Sanford, D. (1989). *Maria's grandma gets mixed up*. Portland, OR: Multnomah.

Selye, H. (1976). *The stress of life* (Rev. ed.). New York: McGraw–Hill.

Severo, R. (1985). *Lisa H*. New York: Harper & Row.

Shute, J. (1992). *Life-size*. New York: Houghton Mifflin.

Stewart, J. (1989). *The body's memory*. New York: St. Martin's Press.

Stone, J. (1980a). "He makes a house call." In J. Stone, *In all this rain* (p. 4). Baton Rouge, LA: Louisiana State University Press.

Stone, J. (1980b). "The girl in the hall." In J. Stone, *In all this rain* (p. 40). Baton Rouge, LA: Louisiana State University Press.

Styron, W. (1990). *Darkness visible*. New York: Random House.

12

Interpersonal Communication

Welcome to the "Information Age!" It is now possible to send and receive messages via electronic mail, voice mail, and along the Internet without ever speaking to another human being. Despite these dramatic advances in communications technology, it is not unusual to hear individuals describe significant problems with interpersonal communication. "He just doesn't listen to me," "I can't talk to my parents," and "She never stops talking," are just some of the frustrations that people voice about a process that seems so easy.

Interpersonal communication is much more than conversation. It has been described by some as, "the basic component of human relationships" (Kozier, Erb, & Olivieri, 1991, p. 247), and by others as, "an act of sharing" (Potter & Perry, 1993, p. 310). Communication is, in its truest sense, an attempt to "know" and understand our fellow human beings; to present ourselves to them and to be present for them. Viewed from this perspective, it seems clear that the ability to communicate effectively does not come naturally. It is, in fact, a learned skill that requires understanding of specific strategies, knowledge of self, and sensitivity to others. In addition, it takes time, energy, practice, and patience to learn to communicate in an effective manner.

The practice of professional nursing requires a high level of facility with interpersonal communication so that an effective relationship between the nurse and the patient can be established and maintained. The nurse's ability to communicate also is integral to the sharing of information, interests, and concerns with patients' families and with members of the health care team. In fact, research has demonstrated a lower incidence of patient mortality in situations where nurses and physicians communicate about patients' needs and coordinate their efforts on behalf of patients

(Knaus, 1986). Such a finding supports the significance of ongoing effective communication when interacting with patients.

DEFINITION OF INTERPERSONAL COMMUNICATION

Interpersonal communication is a complex process that involves the sending and receiving of verbal and nonverbal messages to exchange information and feelings. Because the goal of interpersonal communication is mutual understanding of an intended message, the process necessarily involves active participation by the sender as well as the receiver of the message. The participants in this two-way process engage in a "continuous circular flow of energy" (Lindberg, Hunter, & Kruszewski, 1994, p. 309); that is, they exchange roles as the message and the response are received and interpreted. The cycle is not complete until both participants are satisfied that the message has been transmitted and its meaning understood.

PURPOSES OF COMMUNICATION

Human beings use communication to establish and maintain contact with others, to exchange thoughts and feelings, and to express basic needs. Communication is such a universal phenomenon that one of its classic principles posits that it is not possible for human beings not to communicate (Watzlawich, Beavin, & Jackson, 1967). Thus, a simple shrug of the shoulders constitutes communication if it is perceived by another to have some meaning (Lindberg et al., 1994).

In the practice of professional nursing, communication is used primarily to establish the nurse-patient relationship. This relationship provides the context for the caring behaviors and therapeutic interventions of the nurse that assist individuals, families, and communities to achieve well-being. It is built on a foundation characterized by trust, empathy, caring, and a critical balance between the patient's autonomy and the mutual sharing of decision making by the patient and the nurse (Potter & Perry, 1993).

The development of the nurse-patient relationship involves a building process that does not occur automatically. Through the exercise of well-honed communication skills, the nurse creates an environment of trust that fosters the individual's willingness to share "who" they are with the nurse. Once the relationship is established, the nurse continues to use communication to assist the patient to identify health problems, initiate strategies to resolve problems, and find ways to adapt to problems that cannot be resolved. At this point in the relationship, the nurse implements the professional practice roles of advocate, caregiver, counselor, health teacher, and leader, as needed. The effective implementation of these roles requires that the nurse continue to rely on interpersonal communication as the foundation of professional practice.

MODES OF COMMUNICATION

Communication is achieved through the transmission of verbal and nonverbal messages that are exchanged simultaneously throughout the course of the process. Because both modes are critical to the accurate transmission and reception of thoughts and feelings, nurses need to be aware of and attentive to the characteristics of each.

Verbal Communication

Verbal communication includes the use of the spoken and written word, and because individuals choose the words that they use to express themselves, verbal communication is considered a conscious activity. As a result of this conscious aspect, individuals can choose to reveal as little or as much about themselves as they like. The nurse, however, can enhance openness by creating a nurse-patient relationship that is distinguished by confidentiality and trust.

Verbal language reflects the individual's age, developmental level, education, and cultural background. Individuals also vary the tone, rhythm, and pacing of their verbal messages, which in turn, affects the way their messages are perceived. Thus, assessment of verbal communication demands a holistic approach that is open to the unique differences among individuals.

Effective verbal communication is characterized by qualities such as simplicity, brevity, clarity, appropriate timing, and credibility. Nurses need to be attentive to these qualities in their own speech so that the messages transmitted to patients, families, and colleagues are received and interpreted accurately. Indeed, patients have associated stressful events during hospitalization with health professionals' failure to communicate clearly with them or with members of their family (Spees, 1991).

Although current consumers of health care often are well informed about their disease processes and treatment regimens, individuals still describe feeling overwhelmed by the impersonal nature of the health care system. Accordingly, the nurse should provide information simply, briefly, and clearly. This means that complex ideas should be stated in simple terms, explanations should be free of unnecessary technical jargon, and generalizations, ambiguous statements, and stereotypes should be avoided. In addition, examples and demonstrations are helpful as patients and their families attempt to sort through and make sense of information and instructions.

The nurse's sensitivity to timing also will facilitate the patient's ability to receive and understand messages. For example, patients experiencing pain or emotional distress need to be made comfortable before they can attend to explanations or instructions. In addition, the nurse should avoid allowing the "tasks" of nursing to take priority over the patient's needs and interests. Although it is not always possible to rearrange schedules for patient care, individuals will be more attentive if family visits or phone calls home are not interrupted.

Credibility may be the most critical characteristic of effective verbal communication in that it provides a foundation for trust between the nurse and the patient. In order to be credible, the nurse must share accurate information in a knowledgeable and confident manner. The nurse who reads directions while performing a procedure will have difficulty gaining a patient's confidence! Patients are more likely to be open and comfortable with a nurse who is willing to acknowledge personal limitations, and who is consistent and dependable.

Nonverbal Communication

It has been suggested that approximately 85% of communication is nonverbal (Kozier et al., 1991). Sometimes referred to as "body language," nonverbal communication is the use of actions and symbols other than words to transmit messages. It may include such things as facial expressions, eye contact, touch, and body gestures. Arms folded across the chest, falling asleep in class, and creating physical distances between oneself and others are examples of nonverbal behaviors that transmit powerful messages. Because individuals are often unaware of their body language, nonverbal messages tend to reveal more about intended meanings than the words spoken.

Communication via nonverbal messages enables individuals to bridge gaps created by cultural and language barriers, developmental differences, aphasia, deafness, mental dysfunction, and cognitive disability. In addition, nonverbal language can reenforce or contradict verbal messages. For example, the nurse who asks if a patient has an interest in talking and sits by the bed to await the patient's response, is demonstrating body language consistent with the verbal message. In contrast, the nurse who begins to make the bed when the patient indicates an interest in talking, performs a physical action that is inconsistent with the verbal message.

An understanding of the patient's nonverbal communication requires systematic observation and valid interpretation. It also demands that the nurse be aware of personal nonverbal behaviors. Patients often gauge their response or appropriate level of concern by what they perceive the nurse's nonverbal messages convey. For example, the first time a mastectomy dressing is changed it is not unusual for the patient to look at the nurse's face rather than at the wound. If the nurse does not register revulsion, the patient may have the courage to look at the wound herself. This is not to suggest that nurses should or can always control nonverbal language, but they should be aware of their own expressions, and concentrate on conveying acceptance and regard.

Initial impressions of individuals are based frequently on their physical appearance (Lalli–Acosi, 1990). For example, a crisp, well-tailored look conveys a sense of confidence and professionalism and evokes a positive response from others. The nurse should recognize that general physical appearance—including manner of dress, hygiene, condition of skin, hair, and nails, energy level, and posture and gait—communicates a great deal about an individual's physical and emotional well-being. In addition, a change in an individual's physical appearance may communicate cause for concern to an observant nurse. The failure to attend to appearance and hygiene, for example, may indicate a relapse in a patient who experiences periodic episodes of depression, long before other clinical signs are apparent.

Often, individuals are unaware of the messages that their facial expressions convey. Thus, the latter can be a significant source of information about a person's attitudes and feelings. It is important, however, to validate observations before making judgments and decisions based on nonverbal messages communicated through facial expressions. The nurse may learn that the patient who appeared relaxed and comfortable during his wife's visit was actually "masking" his pain to protect her from more concern about his status.

Eye contact can be subtle, such as a quick sideways glance, or overt, such as the insolent stares of a disturbed adolescent. Use of the eyes for nonverbal communication also is culturally determined; thus, it is important, again, to validate messages that an individual appears to be communicating.

Sometimes individuals use hand gestures, along with verbal communication, to emphasize a point or clarify an intended meaning. At other times, the hands may be the only mode of communication; consider, for example, the constant hand-wringing of the anxious individual or the folded hands of the person who appears relaxed and at ease.

Use of the hands to touch another individual is a highly personalized form of nonverbal communication. Touch can be therapeutic when it is used to convey comfort, or nontherapeutic when it is used to intimidate another human being. Individuals' responses to touch can convey a great deal about their perceptions of interpersonal relationships and their willingness to engage in human contact.

Patients' nonverbal messages also are a significant source of information about their attitudes and feelings. The observant nurse, who is careful to validate observations and consider cultural and personal differences among individuals, will have discovered an invaluable tool for gaining understanding of the emotions that underlie patients' behaviors.

FACTORS THAT AFFECT COMMUNICATION

There are a number of individual and environmental factors that affect a person's ability to communicate, as well as the manner in which that person receives and interprets messages from others. The nurse needs to consider these factors when establishing the nurse-patient relationship and generating a plan of care that will address the patient's unique needs.

Age, developmental level, and facility with language are critical factors that should be evaluated on an individual basis. Because individuals do not conform necessarily to established developmental norms, nurses may need to vary their communication patterns to meet the patient's specific needs. For example, the 45-year-old with a mental disability cannot be expected to understand complex explanations. It also is necessary to avoid stereotypes when communicating with children and the elderly. Many chronically ill children are well aware of their status and are active participants in decision making regarding their care. Also, not all elderly persons are hard of hearing, nor do they appreciate being referred to as "Honey."

The impact of sociocultural background on communication patterns cannot be overstated. Culture encompasses learned behaviors, such as degrees and modes of communication, levels of expressiveness, and the effects of gender and roles on communication. The nurse should acknowledge the effect of sociocultural background on personal patterns of communication, and be open to the differences among patients.

An individual's level of physical and emotional well-being also affects the ability to communicate. Pain, sensory and/or motor deficits, fatigue, stress, withdrawal, prescribed medications, and abuse of addictive substances are examples of factors that may impair or distort communication.

When providing care, the nurse may need to enter the individual's "personal space"; that is, the distance that person prefers for interactions with others. The nurse's invasion of this area may cause the patient to feel vulnerable and may prevent the patient from communicating comfortably with the nurse. Once an individual defines this space, the nurse should retreat to a more suitable distance and warn the patient if the boundary has to be breached at another time.

Similarly, the concept of "territoriality" refers to the space that individuals regard as their own. The drive to acquire and maintain territory is inherent in human beings and provides a sense of identity, security, and control (Potter & Perry, 1993). The cramped quarters of an individual hospital unit, or a chair in a crowded out-patient clinic may be an individual's territory during contact with the health care system. The nurse needs to respect this notion of personal territory as a significant factor affecting the individual's ability and willingness to communicate.

Finally, feelings, beliefs, and values are unique to each individual and play a significant role in determining messages that are transmitted through verbal and nonverbal communication. Strong emotions are sometimes difficult for individuals to express, particularly when they are contrary to the feelings of others. For example, patients who have lost hope that they will recover may not be able to express this to family members. The nurse, familiar with the need to observe and interpret nonverbal communication, may be able to function as an advocate for patients and assist them to articulate their true feelings.

In order to establish effective nurse-patient relationships, nurses need to be aware of the myriad factors that influence interpersonal communication. It also is important that nurses recognize the differences among individuals that make their communication patterns unique to them. Through careful assessment, nurses will be able to identify patients' individual responses to these factors and to plan care that is tailored to the patient's specific needs.

STRATEGIES THAT FOSTER COMMUNICATION

Because the ability to communicate effectively is a learned behavior, the nurse needs to become comfortable with strategies that enhance this process. At first, implementation of some of these strategies may seem stilted and unnatural, but with patience and practice many strategies will become part of the nurse's "natural" communication patterns. Those strategies that continue to be difficult for the nurse to implement should be abandoned. Eventually, the nurse should possess a personal style of communication that uses a variety of strategies and that is flexible and adaptable to the individual needs of patients.

Attentive listening is, perhaps, the most critical of the strategies that enhance communication. The nurse who truly listens conveys acceptance and a willingness to be present to the individual. Listening is characterized by behaviors that provide clear indications that the nurse is making every attempt to understand the patient's message. Sitting close to the patient, nodding as the patient speaks, and making frequent but nonintimidating eye contact are examples of listening behaviors that demonstrate the nurse's interest and concern. Verbal responses such as "I'm listening, go on", and "Yes" also will facilitate communication.

A somewhat difficult, but quite effective strategy, is the appropriate *use of silence*. The desire to comfort a distressed individual through words often is an overwhelming urge; however, the comments that are offered frequently are trivial, and they serve to comfort the nurse more than the patient. A purposeful, quiet period offers the nurse the opportunity to observe the patient and enables the patient to reflect on the stressful situation. Silence that is prolonged or intimidating, however, will not be effective and may disrupt the nurse-patient relationship. Thus, the nurse who uses silence as a strategy to foster communication must be able to recognize silent periods that are helpful and avoid those that may damage the process.

Clarifying and *paraphrasing* are strategies that assist the nurse to understand the patient's message accurately. In addition to indicating to the patient that the nurse is listening, these strategies allow patients to "hear" what they have said, and to gain a clearer perspective on their problem. Clarifying is implemented by a comment such as "I'm not sure that I follow"; paraphrasing is repeating the patient's main ideas in different words.

The patient will be encouraged to continue talking and responding when the nurse implements such strategies as *general leads*, *broad statements*, and *open-ended questions*. Each of these strategies encourages elaboration and assists the patient to explore and articulate ideas and feelings. Questions such as "And then what happened?," "Where would you like to begin today?," and "How did you feel when that happened?" are typical of these helpful approaches.

At times, the nurse may need to obtain specific information or have the patient concentrate on a certain point. On such occasions, the precise, required information can be elicited through the use of *closed questions* such as, "When did the pain begin?," and *focusing*, which uses statements such as, "Tell me more about that incident."

Finally, *summarizing* is a useful strategy when bringing a discussion to an end. It allows the nurse to demonstrate that the patient's message was received, and it affords the patient an opportunity to clarify the intended message.

The various strategies that enhance communication serve to facilitate the establishment of the nurse-patient relationship. Thus, nurses need to identify those techniques that they are most comfortable using, implement the techniques in an appropriate manner, and adapt their use to specific patient situations.

BARRIERS TO EFFECTIVE COMMUNICATION

Although it is not likely that a thoughtful nurse would deliberately hurt a patient during communication, there are comments and behaviors that are much less effective than those just described. Often originating from the nurse's personal discomfort with the patient's situation, these techniques function as barriers to the process of communication. The patient may retreat from a nurse who uses such techniques and eventually disengage entirely from the nurse-patient relationship.

Failure to listen may be the most damaging of the barriers to effective communication. Although the nurse may not be aware of the message that is being transmitted to the patient, behaviors such as standing at the patient's door, moving away from the patient, and changing the subject are clear indications that the nurse's attention is not on the patient.

A number of well-intentioned techniques are actually barriers to communication because they belittle patients' knowledge or cause them to doubt their ability to make decisions. Among these are common barriers such as *voicing approval or disapproval, offering advice and personal opinions,* and *agreeing or disagreeing.* In using such techniques, the nurse is offering judgments that reflect personal values rather than encouraging patients to explore their own values.

Patients seek comfort and support from nurses whom they trust and who encourage them to articulate their deepest concerns. The nurse who trivializes those concerns by offering *false reassurance* discourages the patient from further communication and loses an opportunity to offer hope.

Although often well-intentioned, some communication techniques are less effective than others and may even create barriers to interpersonal communication. Because effective communication is so critical to the nurse-patient relationship, nurses need to evaluate the techniques that they use and eliminate those that prevent patients from sharing their thoughts and feelings with them.

EVALUATION OF COMMUNICATION

A process recording is a formal method of evaluation in which the nurse records all that transpires during communication with a patient, including verbal and nonverbal messages. The process then is reviewed and evaluated to ascertain whether or not the purposes of communication were achieved. In today's busy health care system, it is difficult for nurses to find the time needed to evaluate their communications in a formal way. Nonetheless, nurses should find ways to reflect on the communication strategies that they use and evaluate how helpful those strategies have been. Informal methods of evaluation, such as personal reflection on a specific encounter with a patient, or talking with a colleague about techniques that one has tried, are helpful and can be accomplished in a brief period of time.

THE ARTS AND HUMANITIES IN RELATION TO INTERPERSONAL COMMUNICATION

Because interpersonal communication is so critical to nursing and a skill that can be learned, it is incumbent upon nursing faculty to do all that they can to foster students' ability to communicate well. Although there are numerous textbooks and computer software packages available to assist faculty in this endeavor, the use of a variety of examples from among the arts and humanities is suggested here as an alternative to the more traditional approaches to teaching interpersonal communication.

Literature

Novels

The Great Santini (Conroy, 1976) is a poignant study of the negative effects of the inability to communicate about relationships. Bull

Meacham, a career officer in the military, loves his wife and children, but he is unable to express his feelings in a meaningful way or to understand the messages they attempt to communicate to him. The family experiences numerous highs and lows in their pursuit of mutual understanding, but "what might have been" is never achieved because Bull dies in a plane crash.

Faculty could use this short and easy-to-read novel in several ways. As a case study, *The Great Santini* offers substantive data that students could analyze to generate nursing diagnoses related to communication. In addition, the story can be used to assess communication strategies; for example, faculty might ask students to identify strategies used by the various characters and to distinguish therapeutic techniques from nontherapeutic ones.

John Moon, the protagonist in the novel *Of Such Small Differences* (Greenberg, 1988), is blind and deaf. His isolation from those around him is profound until he meets and falls in love with a young actress named Leda. Because Greenberg captures the young man's dreams and frustrations in very telling prose, the reader is able to gain significant insight into a world that few individuals have known. Thus, the triumph of this novel is its ability to offer the experience of multiple sensory deficits in a realistic, albeit vicarious manner.

Students could be asked to describe their responses to John Moon's story and to share their personal feelings about trying to establish a relationship with an individual who is blind and deaf. In order to facilitate students' abilities to think critically, it would be best if faculty allowed them to discover and cite the factors in the story that enabled the young man to emerge from his isolation. Faculty could then encourage further discussion about therapeutic strategies that enhance communication in individuals who have sensory deficits.

Sue Halpern's (1992) *Migrations to Solitude* is a collection of essays that explore human experiences with privacy and solitude. The author addresses such themes as solitary confinement in a prison cell, voluntary solitude in a monastery, the lack of privacy in an intensive care unit, and the invasion of privacy by modern communication technology. Each essay reflects the author's personal observations of and interviews with individuals who have experienced solitude, or the lack of it, in some form.

This provocative book is useful to a discussion of the notions of personal space and territoriality as factors that affect the ability of individuals to communicate. Students might be perplexed, initially, by the convict's comment that his cell offers him a sense of security. However, his statement supports, in a poignant way, what students learn from textbooks about the relationship between personal space and one's sense of identity and security. With faculty guidance, students could then discuss the lack of privacy that the impersonal nature of the health care system generates, and the ways in which nurses can foster patients' trust and sense of security through effective communication.

Children's Stories

In the children's book, *The Magic Moth* (Lee, 1972), a family's ability to communicate in the midst of a crisis enables them to survive a most difficult time. Maryanne is 10 years old and has been sick for a long time with a heart defect. Her younger brother, Mark–O, learns from his father that Maryanne will die soon. The family talks about Maryanne's death in an open manner; there are no secrets among them. The book is neither sentimental, nor is it simplistic.

Because the death of a child evokes strong personal feelings, faculty could encourage students to express their responses to this story by drawing a picture, creating a poem, or writing a brief personal reflection. Some students might be willing to share their "creations"; often the openness of one student encourages others to participate as well. Once the emotional aspect of this story is addressed, the class then could identify the communication techniques that fostered the family's ability to adapt to such a devastating loss.

Faculty also could propose an alternative plot to this story in which the family cannot communicate effectively. For example, "If the parents were *unable* to talk about the loss of their child, what strategies could a nurse suggest and how might they be implemented in such an intimate situation?" In this exercise, students would need to consider factors that affect communication such as emotions, attitudes, family roles, and stress.

Poetry

Two examples from among the many poems of Robert Frost (1969) are especially useful to teaching interpersonal communication.

The poem, "Meeting and Passing," describes the encounter of two individuals who are traveling in different directions along a country road; they stop, speak, and then move on. The poem addresses social interaction as the first step in developing a relationship. Because students often find it difficult to advance from mere social interactions to more therapeutic levels of communication, this poem could provide the impetus for a discussion of how the communication process can be facilitated.

The importance of listening as a strategy to enhance interpersonal communication is emphasized in the poem, "A Time to Talk" (Frost, 1969). In this very brief work, the narrator asserts that when a friend wants to talk, he puts aside his work and takes time to listen. A parallel can be drawn between this poem and the task-oriented environment in which nursing is practiced. Students could be asked to identify the listening behaviors that are described in the poem, and comment on their importance to effective communication. They also may wish to share how they do or do not attend to listening in their personal and professional relationships. Faculty can foster this discussion by sharing personal experiences with listening, or not listening, to patients and students.

Film and Television

The film, *Children of a Lesser God* (1986), takes place in a school for the deaf, and stars Marlee Matlin, a hearing-impaired actress. Essentially, the film focuses on the relationship that develops between James Leeds, a teacher at the school, and Sarah Norman, an intelligent but isolated young graduate of the school who works there as a janitor. The two fall in love but their relationship is strained by the teacher's attempts to force Sarah to learn to speak. Finally, the two learn to "listen" to each other and in so doing reach a common ground for their relationship. The film is a realistic portrayal of an individual's struggle to be understood, despite the presence of profound physical and emotional barriers to communication. The film also emphasizes the need for human beings to maintain a balance between autonomy and mutual sharing when involved in an interpersonal relationship.

Faculty might find this film useful when teaching the importance of interpersonal communication in the development of the nurse-patient relationship. Scenes from *Children of a Lesser God* should facilitate students' understanding of the barriers that individuals—nurses and patients—can affect to slow this process. Students could be instructed to identify some of the barriers portrayed in the film and to suggest alternative approaches to enhance communication.

The medium of television offers an almost endless supply of resources for nursing faculty who are teaching the concept of interpersonal communication. In addition, television provides the opportunity for students to compare and contrast communication strategies using the many programs that are based on similar formats, such as talk shows and news broadcasts.

One assignment could require that students compare the interviewing techniques of Geraldo Rivera with those of Oprah Winfrey, indicate which approach seemed more effective in eliciting responses, and list the factors that influenced their choice. In a similar assignment, students could be instructed to observe the communication style of news anchor Dan Rather, and assess his verbal messages for clarity, brevity, and credibility. Soap operas and situation comedies could serve as interesting case studies of a variety of difficulties with interpersonal communication. Being assigned to watch several sequences of a program to gather assessment data would not be an undue burden because many students already have a "favorite show" that they manage to view around their class schedule.

Finally, the ever-present product advertisements on commercial television are useful to foster students' awareness of effective verbal communication. For the most part, these interruptions in programming are brief, clear, and concise. They have precious few minutes in which to achieve their goal of convincing viewers to buy a certain product. Students could identify those ads that use clear, concise language and contrast them with ads that are more obscure. This exercise could emphasize the relationship between the use of clear, concise language and the successful transmission of an important message.

Fine Arts

Drama

The compelling story of Helen Keller was captured beautifully in William Gibson's 1959 play, *The Miracle Worker*. Blind and deaf, the child, Helen, lived in a world characterized by fear, isolation, and frustration until her parents hired Annie Sullivan to be her teacher. Through persistence, and despite almost overwhelming odds, Annie overcame Helen's resistance to her and taught Helen how to function as an independent human being. The play underscores the importance of such basic skills of interpersonal communication as perseverance, flexibility, self-knowledge, and the willingness to recognize the uniqueness of individuals.

In an ideal situation students would have the opportunity to experience a live performance of this play. Occasionally, college and/or community theater groups recreate this classic drama, and it is well worth investigating such a possibility. The play, however, was adapted for film, under the same title, and is available on videocassette. Thus, faculty can preview the film and show selected segments in class as a means of introducing the topic of communication strategies. Students may remember this graphic portrayal of interpersonal communication long after their reading from the textbook is forgotten.

Music

Because the process of communication is not complete until both the sender and the receiver share a mutual understanding of the intended message, nurses need to communicate in a clear and precise manner. The song, "Hello, Goodbye," written by John Lennon and Paul McCartney, challenges listeners to consider how they use words and how their ideas and feelings are perceived by others (Bruderle, 1994). In addition, this musical piece, with its playful melody and repetitive lyrics, is a welcome addition to a discussion about the need for nurses to accept the ideas and feelings of patients and to recognize that agreeing/disagreeing and approving/disapproving actually function as barriers to effective communication.

The effect of past experiences on the ability to communicate with others and establish meaningful relationships with them is depicted poignantly in Paul Simon's "I Am a Rock." Simon and Garfunkel sing of an individual who has withdrawn to a safe place where no one can hurt him or get close to him and where he does not have to reach out to others. The individual has built "walls" for protection and declares he is strong and can stand alone.

This song offers insight regarding the risks inherent in forming interpersonal relationships, and the tactics that individuals use to avoid significant contact with others. In addition, faculty can use

this song to address the need for nurses to understand the underlying motivations that affect human behavior.

The inner longings of a deaf, mute, and blind, 9-year-old boy are
expressed clearly in the song, "See Me, Feel Me," from the popular
rock opera, "Tommy," written by Peter Townshend and The Who.
The song provides insight into an individual's pursuit of human
understanding, insight that could never be detailed adequately in
a textbook. Thus, students have the opportunity to gain empathic
awareness of the inability to communicate and to express that
awareness in their caring relationships with patients.

Students may wish to describe their initial feelings on hearing
this song before discussing its clinical application. Perhaps faculty
could list students' feelings on the board as a way of helping them
recognize the different ways that individuals respond to the same
stimulus and acknowledge that all these reactions are legitimate.

Faculty also could suggest this song to members of a clinical
group who are assigned to present a postconference. Imagine the
impact on the rest of the group if the students used this piece to
introduce their discussion of impaired verbal communication.
Perhaps the students would find it easier to suggest realistic and
appropriate communication strategies if they were to respond to
the situation presented through a song rather than through a clinical case study.

Painting

One of the advantages of interpersonal communication is that it
enables individuals to share in the simple pleasure of each others'
company. The delightful painting, "The Friendly Call" by William
Chase, depicts two young women pleasantly engaged in quiet conversation. They represent an era when women wore long dresses
and spent leisurely afternoons discussing pleasant matters. The
women are focused on each other and they appear comfortable
and at ease. Although there is a marked contrast between the life
style of the young women in this painting and that of the current
culture, the ease at communication that is obvious is, nonetheless,
timely and appealing.

This painting could serve as a starting point for a discussion
about the appropriate environment for effective interpersonal
communication. Students could be instructed to identify factors in
the scene that facilitate communication; it is hoped that students

would note such factors as privacy, timing, comfort, and physical closeness. Students also could describe the settings in which they encounter patients and the effects of these settings on patients' willingness to share their ideas and feelings.

Faculty seeking ways to enliven an introductory class on interpersonal communication could begin by asking students to share their personal experiences of not being listened to by others. "How do you feel when you realize that no one is listening to you?" is an excellent trigger question. Students who choose to respond to this question may describe such feelings as anger, frustration, indifference, and loneliness. Unfortunately, it will not be unlikely that several students will have similar experiences to share.

At this point, faculty could display Andrew Wyeth's painting, "Wind from the Sea," and ask students to contrast their perceptions of this work with the feelings about listening that were shared previously. The painting depicts an open window through which blows a gentle breeze from the sea. The view from the window centers on the sea beyond and an open road that leads to the water. "Wind from the Sea" is an ideal metaphor for the benefits of effective interpersonal communication in that it portrays openness, clarity, and unity. Although students may need encouragement at first, faculty should refrain from influencing students' perceptions. Students need to acquire knowledge by manipulating information and experiences in their own unique manner.

The artist Degas depicted life in a most realistic manner. "L'Absinthe," a classic example of his artistic approach, is a study of the isolation that two people can experience despite being seated next to each other. The woman's physical appearance communicates a sense of loneliness; her body is drooped and her facial expression is sad. The man's apparent indifference to her is evident in his bland facial expression and his failure to turn in her direction.

The painting provides a focal point for a discussion of the importance of stating observations as a therapeutic communication technique. Although the woman certainly appears to be in some distress, the man's role is not clear. Faculty could ask students why they think the woman looks so sad, or how they would respond if they came upon a similar situation in a clinical setting. A role-play exercise, in which students "become" the characters in the painting, could be an effective way for students to respond to these questions. Students also may recognize, as a result of their classmates' role-playing, that initial perceptions need validation.

Sculpture

Rodin's sculpture, "The Thinker," is a familiar work of art that depicts a man in an introspective pose. The man is leaning forward and his hand rests on his chin. His body language appears to reflect deep thought, and his youthful appearance suggests great physical strength. Although this work portrays a sense of silence, it is, indeed, highly communicative.

This work could be used to introduce the ways that individuals communicate and to emphasize the need for nurses to attend to patients' nonverbal messages. In addition, it could serve as a springboard for a discussion of the relationship between verbal and nonverbal communication and the need for nurses to identify and address incongruent messages from patients, such as the patient who appears pensive but is experiencing significant physical pain or inner turmoil.

CONCLUSION

Interpersonal communication, like nursing, is both an art and a science. It requires an awareness of certain principles and an understanding of the uniqueness of human expressions of ideas and feelings. Learning to communicate in an effective manner is not easy, but because it is the basis of the nurse-patient relationship, it is a critical nursing skill. Textbooks do offer much information about the mechanics of interpersonal communication, but rarely do they address the humanistic aspect. The arts and humanities integrated into nursing education in a thoughtful manner may fill that gap and enable students to communicate in a more effective manner.

REFERENCES

Bruderle, E. (1994). The arts and humanities: A creative approach to developing nurse leaders. *Holistic Nursing Practice, 9*(1), 68–74.

Conroy, P. (1976). *The great Santini.* Boston: Houghton Mifflin.

Frost, R. (1969). *The poetry of Robert Frost.* New York: Holt, Rinehart and Winston.

Greenberg, J. (1988). *Of such small differences*. New York: Henry Holt and Company.

Halpern, S. (1992). *Migrations to solitude*. New York: Pantheon.

Knaus, W. A. (1986). An evaluation of outcomes from intensive care units in major medical centers. *Annals of Internal Medicine, 104,* 410.

Kozier, B., Erb, G., & Olivieri, R. (1991). *Fundamentals of nursing* (4th ed.). Redwood City, CA: Addison–Wesley.

Lalli–Acosi, S. (1990). Polishing your self-image. *Healthcare Trends and Transitions, 1*(2), 15.

Lee, V. (1972). *The magic moth*. New York: Seabury.

Lindberg, J., Hunter, M., & Kruszewski, A. (1994). *Introduction to nursing* (2nd ed.). Philadelphia: Lippincott.

Potter, P., & Perry, A. (1993). *Fundamentals of nursing* (3rd ed.). St. Louis, MO: Mosby.

Spees, C. (1991). Knowledge of medical terminology among patients and families. *Image: Journal of Nursing Scholarship, 23,* 225–229.

Watzlawich, P., Beavin, J., & Jackson, D. (1967). *Pragmatics of human communication*. New York: Norton.

13

Leadership

Leadership is a complex phenomenon which has been studied and written about extensively. It has been the focus of countless research studies, the topic of numerous books and articles, the theme of extensive numbers of conferences and presentations, and a goal of many academic programs including those in nursing. But despite this attention over a number of decades, leadership continues to be confused with management, and it remains "one of the least understood phenomenon on earth" (Burns, 1978, p. 2). In fact, after analyzing "a century of leadership research," VanFleet & Yukl (1989, p. 66) concluded, "where once we thought of leadership as a relatively simple construct, we now recognize that it is among the more complex social phenomena."

When we think of leaders and leadership, we frequently call to mind presidents, prime ministers, CEOs, academic deans, and others in positions of authority. And we often fail to acknowledge the importance of followers in the success of leaders. This discussion will explore the nature of leadership and the characteristics or qualities of effective leaders, distinguish between leadership and management, and examine the role of followers. Various art forms will then be proposed as means to assist nursing students to understand this important concept.

THE NATURE OF LEADERSHIP

Leadership is a multifaceted concept and a universal phenomenon. Whether we interact with others in the home, on the playground, in organizations, in corporate offices, in the political arena, in the halls of academe, or in our local communities, the potential for leadership to be exercised exists. Whenever several people come together, particularly if they need to solve a problem, formulate a strategy, or set a direction, leadership is likely to be exercised. But what is this elusive, ambiguous phenomenon, and why do we need to be concerned about it?

Bennis and Nanus (1985) noted that, "If there was ever a moment in history when a comprehensive strategic view of leadership was needed, ... this is certainly it" (p. 2). Ours is a world characterized by constant change, uncertainty, unpredictability, unprecedented ethical dilemmas, explosions in knowledge and information, and heightened interdependence. Leadership is needed to chart a strong course through this turmoil and to help individuals, groups, organizations, and communities emerge from it with strength and focus.

Leadership involves articulating a vision, communicating that vision to others in such a way that they choose to follow in its pursuit, and mobilizing others to work toward realization of the vision. It is the pivotal force behind successful groups and organizations, and it provides the focus and the energy to create a preferred future.

As an art more than a science, leadership means "liberating people to do what is required of them, in the most effective and humane way possible" (DePree, 1989, p. 1). It is "more tribal than scientific . . . more a weaving of relationships than an amassing of information" (p. 3). But despite it being an art, experts (DePree, 1989; Gardner, 1990) assert leadership can be learned—at least some of the elements of leadership can be learned.

If it is to be exercised, leadership requires leaders. Leaders are people who have vision, an ability to express the vision, commitment or passion, and energy and enthusiasm. They use intuition and common sense, are willing to dream dreams and attempt the impossible, take risks, dislike the status quo, engage in introspection, are self-confident, pursue excellence, and, in the words of Winston Churchill, "Never, never, never quit!"

"No man or woman becomes a leader unless he or she wants to. They've got to have a burning need to get there" (Ludlum, 1988, p. 264). Thus, leaders have to be so driven by their vision that it becomes a fire burning inside, a passion that guides what they do.

Consider Martin Luther King and his long struggle for civil rights and racial equality. Every ounce of his being was devoted to these goals, and he risked and endured imprisonment and ridicule for them. He even risked his life and died for these goals. There is no doubt, as one reads or listens to his "I Have a Dream" speech, that he was passionate about the equality of all people. Martin Luther King was, without question, a leader.

Candy Lightner was so enraged with "the system" after the loss of her daughter in 1980 to a drunk driver, that she formed Mothers Against Drunk Drivers (MADD). MADD is now a nationwide organization that educates the public about the dangers of drinking and driving, campaigns and lobbies to keep drunk drivers off our roads, and advocates for appropriate punishment of those who violate these laws. Candy Lightner was not an elected public official or a CEO of a Fortune 500 company. She was an individual with a vision of a safer world, especially for children, she communicated that vision to others, and she acted, in cooperation with others who chose to follow in that cause, with passion and focus. She was a leader.

And consider Eleanor Roosevelt. She was the wife of a well-known, powerful figure, and she could have gone through life enjoying the benefits of her status, wealth, and fame. But Eleanor Roosevelt was not content to sit back and merely fulfill the social functions of a First Lady (Goodwin, 1994). Indeed, she was a social activist who traveled the country and the world, working to improve the life of the poor, the unemployed, laborers, and other groups often ignored or neglected by society. Throughout her life, Eleanor Roosevelt worked for a more humanitarian society and served as a true leader in helping make that vision a reality.

These are but a few examples of individuals who have taken on the challenge of leadership. They demonstrate the essence of what leadership is, as well as what it is not. Leadership is not merely being the center, nucleus, or head of a group. It is not forcing others to comply with some rule or policy. It is not the abuse of power. And it is not merely saying what others want to hear and maintaining the status quo.

Leadership can be thought of in terms of certain qualities or characteristics of an individual. Indeed, research (Bass, 1990) has shown positive correlations with leadership and the following traits: above-average height and/or weight, an abundant reserve of energy, cooperativeness, tactfulness, a higher degree of education, superior judgment, decisiveness, verbal fluency, venturesomeness, persistence, a sense of personal identity, and a readiness to absorb interpersonal stress.

Leadership also has been conceptualized in terms of tasks to be performed on a short-term, as well as long-term, basis, and with individuals, as well as with an entire group. The tasks of leadership (Gardner, 1989, 1990) have been identified as follows:

Envisioning Goals . . . pointing others in the right direction and dealing with the tension between long- and short-term goals

Affirming Values . . . revitalizing the beliefs and values shared by those in the group

Motivating . . . knowing individuals in the group, having and promoting positive attitudes, and encouraging others to be excited about the future and how they can be a part of it

Managing . . . planning, setting priorities, and making decisions

Achieving a Workable Unity . . . building a sense of community in the group, "creating loyalty to the larger venture" (Gardner, 1989, p. 29), and working toward cohesion

Explaining . . . helping members of the group understand what the goal is, why they are being asked to do certain things, and how their work relates to "the big picture"

Serving as a Symbol . . . acting as the group's source of unity, voice of anger, collective identity, and hope

Representing the Group . . . speaking and acting for or on behalf of the group to external constituencies

Renewing . . . breaking routines, habits, fixed attitudes, perceptions, and assumption; keeping "a measure of diversity and dissent in the system [as a way to avoid] the trance of nonrenewal" (Gardner, 1989, p. 33)

It is obvious from this discussion that leadership is not easy, and it "is not tidy" (Gardner, 1989, p. 33). It also is obvious that leadership is not the same as management.

LEADERSHIP AND MANAGEMENT

Although the terms often are used interchangeably in the literature, leadership and management are distinct concepts. The seminal work of Zaleznik (1977) in this area, and subsequent work by Moloney (1979), Rost (1985), Bennis (1989a), and Manfredi and Valiga (1990) are useful in distinguishing these related but different phenomena.

Management must be understood as a position, a particular role in an organization. Leadership, on the other hand, may or not be exercised through a position of authority in an organization. In fact, in light of the preceding discussion about leaders being "boat rockers" and disliking the status quo, one might conclude that it may be easier to be a true leader if one were *not* tied to a position of authority!

Leaders relate to others through influence, whereas managers relate to others through authority. Managers' employees are expected to obey legitimate authority, but leaders have followers who attach themselves informally and who are under no compulsion to obey orders. Such individuals *choose* to follow a leader because they believe the leader can clearly articulate goals and outline ways to achieve those goals which they, the followers, support and in which they believe.

As noted, leaders have a vision that motivates their actions and causes them to be willing to be leaders in the first place. The vision they have is their cause or their purpose in life, and they are willing to expend enormous amounts of energy on it. This vision is value driven, resulting in leaders being more concerned with ends than with processes. Managers, on the other hand, are— and, indeed, need to be—motivated by organizational objectives. They see themselves as problem solvers who work to see that the organization's goals are reached. They are concerned with process-es, and they detail those processes (through policies, etc.) careful-ly. In essence, "managers are people who do things right and leaders are people who do the right thing" (Bennis & Nanus, 1985, p. 21).

Leaders are change agents, innovators who prize their ability to keep groups or organizations moving ahead and the people in them searching for new ways of doing things better. They take risks and are comfortable with alterations in the status quo. Managers, by comparison, strive to maintain organizations and change them only incrementally. They are low-risk takers who try to avoid high-risk, potentially counterproductive behaviors.

Associated with the degree of comfort with change is the degree of comfort with conflict. Leaders are comfortable with conflict, seek it out or even introduce it, and use it to achieve their objec-tives. Managers, in contrast, try to control conflict; they try to resolve conflict situations so that the conflict is managed, meaning it is kept at an acceptable, minimal level, or it is eliminated.

Additionally, leaders use intuition in making decisions, they are more comfortable with ambiguity, and they are creative; they want to see new forms take shape, new ideas develop, and new goals fulfilled. By comparison, managers are more inclined to engage in rational decision making, to be more comfortable with predictability, and to be more adept at taking a project that has already been conceptualized by someone else and regulating resources and activities so that the project can be a success.

Finally, managers have a more practical bent and an external locus of control. Leaders, in contrast, have an intellectual frame of reference and an internal locus of control.

Zaleznik's (1977) work helps summarize some of the distinctions between leaders and managers. He asserted that managers are problem solvers who emphasize rationality and control. They adopt impersonal attitudes toward goals, accepting those espoused by an organization; they dislike and avoid solitary activity and prefer to work with people; and they are what he called "once-born" individuals, those "whose lives have more or less been a peaceful flow from the moment of their births" (Zaleznik, 1977, p. 72). Managers work to perpetuate existing institutions.

Leaders, on the other hand, are imaginative and are driven by ideas and possibilities, not assurances. They create their own goals in conjunction with the group and are highly invested in those goals; they are more empathic toward people, concerned with the meaning that events and decisions have for people; and they are comfortable with solitary activity since it provides time for reflection and dreaming. Leaders are what Zaleznik (1977, p. 72) called "twice-born" personalities, whose "lives are marked by a continual struggle." In essence, leaders work *in* organizations but never belong *to* them.

Table 13.1 summarizes some of the differences between leaders and managers. A word of caution, however. When reviewing the table and reflecting on the preceding discussion, it is important to keep in mind that extremes have been used to illustrate the differences between leadership and management. Without doubt, there are many managers who are providing leadership in their units, their organizations, or the committees they chair. But not all managers are leaders automatically or by default. In fact, "we follow to the fullest when leadership is based on expertness or an admirable goal, not because of a title or organizational status" (Kelley, 1992, p. 9).

TABLE 13.1 Summary of Differences between Leaders and Managers

MANAGER	LEADER
Engages in activities of efficiency	Engages in activities of vision and judgment
Excels in ability to handle daily routines	Questions whether the routines should be done at all
Optimizes the present state affairs	Wants to create a new state of affairs
Does not like surprises	Likes surprises
Tied to a designated position in an organizationan	Free standing and not limited to organizational position
Once born	Twice born
Administers	Innovates
A copy	An original
Maintains	Develops
Focuses on systems and structures	Focuses on people
Relies on control	Inspires trust
Short-range view	Long-range perspective
Asks how and when	Asks what and why
Has her eye on the bottom line	Has her eye on the horizon
Imitates	Originates
Accepts the status quo	Challenges the status quo
A "good soldier"	Her "own person"
Does things right	Does the right thing
Wears a "square hat"	Wears a sombrero
Learns through training	Opts for true education
Solves problems	Finds problems
Surrenders to the context	Masters the context
Prefers to work with others	Enjoys solitary activity
Acts to limit choices	Creates opportunities and excitement
Adopts an impersonal attitude toward goals	Adopts a personal and active attitude toward goals
An eventful person (whose actions influence change)	An event-making person (whose actions create a new future)
Concerned primarily with achieving organizational goals	May be working for goals that have no direct relation to the organization
Emphasizes rationality and control	Seems to generate relative disorder
Is appointed	Is chosen freely by followers

Primary sources used by T. Valiga to develop this compilation:

Bennis, W. (1989). *On becoming a leader*. Reading, MA: Addison–Wesley.

Zaleznik, A. (1977). Manager and leaders: Are they different? *Harvard Business Review, 55*(3), 67–78.

In addition, and perhaps more important, it is critical to note that not all leaders are managers. Candy Lightner did not start out as the head of MADD. Martin Luther King did not start out as the head of the Southern Christian Leadership Conference, an organization with the aim of "seek[ing] reconciliation and the formation of a community based on love . . . the beloved community" (Ansbro, 1982, p. 197). Nelson Mandela did not start out as President of South Africa. And Florence Nightingale did not start out as "the founder of modern nursing." One does not have to be in a position of authority to provide leadership. But what one does need is followers.

THE ART OF FOLLOWERSHIP

One would assume that most people would prefer to be thought of as leaders rather than followers. The role of follower, historically, has been given little attention in discussions of and research about leadership, and the role often is viewed as distasteful.

Followers often are thought of as passive, mindless, dependent individuals who have no status and no significant role in affecting change. In reality, however, effective followers have the same characteristics as leaders, they are (or should be considered as) cohorts of (Brown, 1980) or collaborators with (Rost, 1994) the leader, and they are as important as the leader in the relationship. In fact, they may be even more important in the relationship since leaders can be leaders only if they have followers!

Leaders may create new ideas, but it is the followers who test those ideas. Leaders inspire vision, and followers supply the energy to achieve that vision. Leaders may make decisions, but followers are the ones who challenge those decisions. Leaders create environments of trust and freedom, and followers must use that freedom responsibly if goals are to be achieved and visions realized. Both leaders and followers take risks, both must know themselves, both must be trustworthy and respectful, and both must be willing to work collaboratively with others. Thus, leaders and followers complement each other and reflect many similar traits (Corona, 1986).

There is a reciprocal relationship or an interdependence that exists between effective leaders and effective followers. Each stimulates, reinforces, challenges, and supports the other, and they enter into a partnership. There is an intimacy and a personal "covenental relationship" (DePree, 1989, p. 60) between leaders and followers. In other words, "leaders and followers are a rhythm" (Malone, 1990).

Unfortunately, however, not all followers are effective. Followers can sabotage the efforts of the leader, they can create unrest in the group, and they can be apathetic and fail to give leaders the critical feedback leaders need. Ineffective followers can be uncommitted and unwilling to participate, hostile, or chronically tired and angry; or they can consistently convey a negative or "it-can-never-work" attitude.

Various types of followers are addressed thoroughly by Kelley (1989, 1992) and summarized in Figure 13.1. "Sheep" are people who are easily led and manipulated, as was the case with the Jim Jones cult in Guyana, where over 300 people committed mass suicide at his urging. Sheep are passive, dependent, fail to think critically about the leader's actions or the direction in which the group is headed, take no responsibility, and never take risks.

FIGURE 13.1   Types of Followers . . . Followership Styles

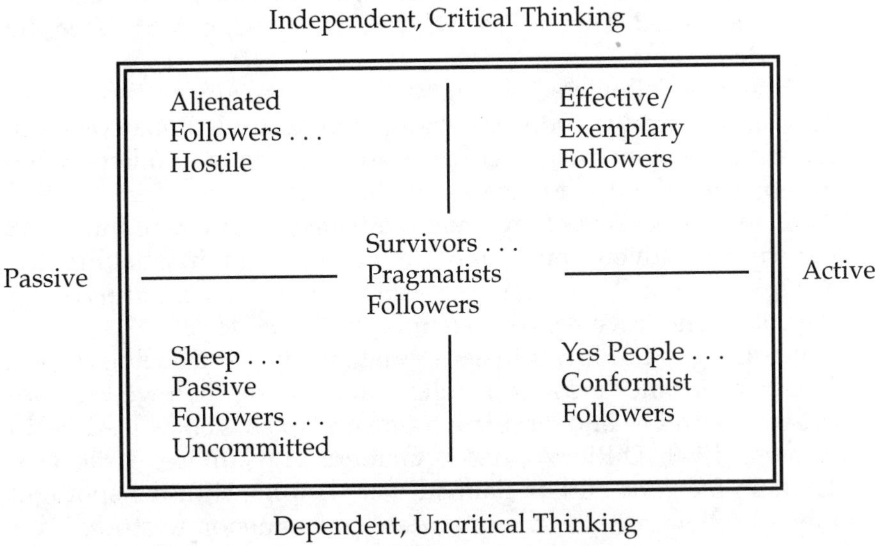

Independent, Critical Thinking

Alienated Followers . . . Hostile		Effective/ Exemplary Followers
Passive ———————	Survivors . . . Pragmatists Followers	——————— Active
Sheep . . . Passive Followers . . . Uncommitted		Yes People . . . Conformist Followers

Dependent, Uncritical Thinking

"Yes people" also fail to engage in critical thinking, ask questions, or think for themselves. Unlike sheep, however, they are active participants in the organization and carry out the leader's directives, often with enthusiasm. Oliver North in the Iran–Contra scandal or many of Hitler's cabinet members are examples of this type of follower.

Another type of ineffective follower is the "Alienated Follower." Unlike the relatively mindless type just discussed, Alienated Followers do think critically about things happening around them and, perhaps, affecting them directly; however, they are not motivated to act on the insights gained from such critical thinking. They remain passive, withdrawn and hostile, and while they may sabotage the effects of the leader, they do so in a subtle way. "Hawkeye Pierce, in the TV series *MASH*, personified the 15% to 25% of followers who are alienated" (Kelley, 1992, p. 100).

"Pragmatists" are middle-of-the-road followers. They will question, but will not be too critical. They will not take a strong position on controversial issues or stick their necks out, and they are happy to do what is required of them, keep a low profile, and not get too involved. They follow what Kelley (1992, p. 118) called the "agenda du jour."

"Effective Followers," in contrast, are independent, think carefully and critically about the group's goals and directions, give feedback and constructive criticism to the leader and others in the group, play devil's advocate, are innovative and creative, and think for themselves. They are good team players, take initiative, participate actively, and want to be involved in shaping the group's agenda. They share the leader's commitment to realizing the vision and have a passion similar to the leader's.

Being a good follower takes special talents just as being a good leader does. Since most of us follow much more than we lead, we need to attend to and cultivate followership as well as leadership (Brown, 1980; DiRienzo, 1994; Guidera & Gilmore, 1988; Lee, 1993). In fact, one author claimed that "helping shift the spotlight toward followership is the important phenomenon to study if we are to understand why organizations succeed or fail" (Kelley, 1992, p. 5).

There is no doubt that leadership is hard work. And because of this, we often lament the lack of leadership in our society. We see reference made to "the debris of leaders" (Bennis, 1989b, p. 6) and suggestions that leaders are an "endangered species" (Bennis, 1989b, p. 5). We read criticisms about our school leaders, political leaders, religious leaders, business leaders, and organizational leaders, and we note that they fail to move us forward in healthy, positive directions. This may be so. But one also must examine the role of followers in the process of moving forward and question whether they have done all they could do to be effective followers.

Barbara Barnum (1987) wrote in a commentary that a field sometimes "needs a hero or a bunch of heros, an elite to set its course, to chart new lands, to brave new worlds" (p. 5). However, in this increasingly complex and ever-changing world, the course these heros often must chart, noted Barnum, is an extremely difficult one. Under these circumstances, it is the *followers* who must be brave men and women, and it may be the heros—the leaders—who "may have the easiest job of it" (p. 5).

REFLECTIONS ON LEADERSHIP

According to the futurists Naisbitt and Aburdene (1990), "we stand at the dawn of a new era" (p. 11), an era characterized by constant change, increased interdependence, a broader world view, heightened ambiguity and uncertainty, and greater demands for accountability. Such an era will be navigated successfully only through the combined efforts of competent leaders and effective, exemplary, enlightened followers.

We can no longer fail to attend to the cultivation and development of followership skills. We can no longer afford to confuse leadership with management. And we can no longer administer "the antileadership vaccine" (Gardner, 1993) which inhibits or interferes with the development of people as leaders.

Gardner (1993) asserted that we administer the "antileadership vaccine" when we allow people to remain anonymous, blend into the background, fail to take a stand on things in which they believe, or fail to act. We also fail to prepare leaders for tomorrow when we emphasize narrow, rather than broad, views and when we fail to help people see just what leadership is. Perhaps through the use of the arts and humanities, nursing students can be helped to understand the true nature of leadership, the relationships that need to exist between leaders and followers, and how they can begin to take responsibility as effective followers and eventually effective leaders. As noted, the arts and humanities foster self-reflection, individual interpretations, and an appreciation of different perspectives; as such, they would seem to be particularly useful in helping students learn about the complex concept, leadership.

THE ARTS AND HUMANITIES IN RELATION TO LEADERSHIP

Since leadership is such a multidimensional phenomenon that has relevance in all aspects of life, the resources available to nurse educators to help students learn about this concept are extensive. One need only be open to the many possibilities.

Literature

Novels

An excellent literary source to use in a study of leadership styles and leader-follower relationships is the classic novel *Watership Down* (Adams, 1972). This is a story about a group of rabbits who leave their warren in search of a safer place. Along their journey, they encounter other groups of rabbits, participate in several existing warrens, and create their own community. Throughout this tale, the reader has the opportunity to see an authoritarian, a laissez faire, a totalitarian, and a democratic leader "in action," appreciate the effect the leader's style has on the followers, and realize the different strengths individuals have and how each can emerge as a leader in different circumstances. All of these insights are relevant to the study of leadership. Although there is an animated film version of this book, it does not convey the leadership concepts as well; thus, it is suggested that students read the novel, after being given adequate time and clear directions on what to look for as they read (e.g., leadership types and the leader-follower interactions), and after they have been "warned" not to let themselves become too frustrated with the "rabbit-ese" language used throughout.

Machiavelli's *The Prince* (1966) also might be considered by nurse educators as a resource to facilitate an understanding of leadership or, perhaps more accurately, "what *not* to do if you hope to be an effective leader in this day and age." Written in 16th century Italy, when treachery was a strategy needed for survival in many royal courts, this little book often is cited as an illustration of the abuse of power. Leaders have power, power they derive from their knowledge, hierarchial position, networks with significant others, or other sources, and power they can abuse or use effectively. After reading *The Prince*, students could be asked to examine the behaviors of those in positions of authority in terms of their bases of power, their effective use of power, the ways in which they empower others, or their abuse of power, either obviously or subtly. It is doubtful they would find someone as extreme as Machiavelli described, but the abuse of power occurs in many subtle ways, and students would do well to reflect on that regarding others' behaviors and their own.

Another excellent source for studying leadership is biographies of individuals in our past or contemporary world. Works about Abraham Lincoln, John F. Kennedy, Margaret Sanger, Eleanor Roosevelt, Gandhi, Nelson Mandela, Winston Churchill, and many others can serve to introduce students to some of the great thinkers and leaders of our times and help them appreciate the ordinary beginnings of many of these people. Biographies also document the passions and visions of the person under study, as well as their sustained work to turn their dreams into realities.

Finally, although it is not a novel, *The Bible* can be thought of as an example in this category and used as an illustration of the leadership style, characteristics, and effectiveness of Jesus Christ. Many stories in *The Bible* convey Christ's vision of an established Kingdom of God where peace and justice prevail, His ability to communicate that vision in ways the multitudes could understand, and His untiring efforts to convey the message to all who would listen. They also reveal Christ's ability to "wake people up," relate effectively to others, trust His apostles enough that they were encouraged to spread the word, understand the needs and fears of those being asked to follow, and live a life that warranted others' trust. All of these behaviors are consistent with those of leaders, and all these and more could be gleaned by students from reading *The Bible*.

Short Stories and Children's Stories

Leadership styles, and perhaps the difference between leadership and management, also might be gleaned from Aesop's fable, *The Sun and the Wind*. In this story, the sun and the wind challenge each other to see who can remove the cloak of a traveler on the road.

The wind uses force, which might be likened to rigid rules, policies, coercion and power abuse; the effect is that the traveler, who might be thought of as an employee, pulls his cloak even tighter around himself and withdraws into himself. The sun, on the other hand, uses warmth and heat, which might be likened to encouragement, support, open communication, honesty, and empowerment; the effect is that the traveler, who might be conceptualized as an effective follower, removes his cloak, and the sun's goal is achieved. One can conclude that kindness and gentleness often are more influential than force and a dictatorial approach.

Students also can learn a great deal about effective leaders from the writings of the 6th century B.C. Chinese statesman and philosopher, Lao-tzu. In particular, his *Tao Te Ching* (Mitchell, 1988) is a useful resource. This is a collection of 81 chapters, each a single page long or less, and many offering sage advice for aspiring leaders. Included among these writings are suggestions for leaders to let group members have some control over destiny and not intervene unless it is necessary, have a sense of self, be grounded and know where they stand, have integrity, and help others find their own success. Students could be asked to reflect on one or several chapters, discuss the main idea in each, and discuss the relevance of that wisdom in today's contemporary world, 2,500 years after the words were written.

The Little Engine That Could (Piper, 1961) is a children's story about a train chugging up a steep mountain out of sheer determination and persistence—"I think I can I think I can"—the kind of drive frequently needed by leaders who "never, never quit" (Churchill) in pursuing their goals and turning their dreams into reality, despite barriers, side tracks, and steep hills. Shel Silverstein's poem, "The Little Blue Engine" (1974), takes this theme even further and notes that "if the track is tough and the hill is rough, [merely] thinking you can just ain't enough!" (p. 158). Students could be asked to look at leaders in nursing's past and present, leaders in fields other than nursing, the nurses on the units with which they affiliate, or their peers to determine what qualities, other than determination and a positive outlook, make them leaders. If "thinking you can just ain't enough," then what is enough?

Another story written primarily for children that has relevance in a study of leadership is *The Velveteen Rabbit* (Williams, 1975), originally written in 1922. This very short story tells of a stuffed rabbit that was owned by a little boy. The rabbit was not fancy and felt insignificant and commonplace among the other toys; however, he did not "put on airs" as many of the other toys did. Instead, he was real and genuine. He develops a reciprocal relationship with the boy and comes to realize that one becomes real when loved by others, and becoming real takes time. This tale could be used to facilitate a discussion of the need for leaders to be genuine, to know and relate well to others if they are to be effective, and to fight the temptations of an easy life when that deflects one from one's vision.

The well-known story of *The Emperor's New Clothes* also could serve as a source of a greater understanding of the concept of leadership. In this tale, the Emperor hires a tailor to fashion him a new set of clothes so that he may walk even more proudly among his people. The tailor spends days supposedly creating the new clothes and repeatedly telling the Emperor that they surely will be elegant and unlike any that he has worn before. Despite these claims, the tailor spends his days lazily doing nothing. Finally, he must present the new clothes to the Emperor, which he does. He walks into the chambers carrying the clothes in a careful fashion and carrying on about how superb they are; the only problem is that his hands are empty. Not wanting to look like a fool and admit that he sees nothing, the Emperor goes along with the charade, commenting that the clothes are, indeed, magnificent and ultimately believing that he sees them! When the day comes for the Emperor to parade through the streets to show off his new clothes, he does so in his underwear; however, no one will tell him that there *are* no new clothes except for one innocent young boy. This story seems to speak to the effects of being so impressed with one's self and one's position of authority that one cannot bear to confront the truth. It also provides an excellent example of ineffective followers who fail to challenge or question the leader, and the potentially disastrous outcome of that kind of inaction. The story can be used as a framework for students to analyze the literature, their nursing colleagues, and themselves in terms of leadership qualities and characteristics, and the extent to which they have functioned as effective followers.

Finally, *The Little Prince* (de Saint–Exupéry, 1943) is a classic tale that could be used by nurse educators. This story tells of a little prince who travels the universe and encounters many people who are self-absorbed; he meets a king whose authority must be obeyed, a lamplighter who blindly follows orders, and others who are impressed with their own importance, but who are all alone. The little prince seeks advice on how to care for the single rose on his planet, a rose he loves dearly. In his quest, he wants to learn, asks many questions, strives to understand others, and is imaginative, creative, and open to all possibilities. He comes to realize the importance of being judged by deeds rather than words, knowing others and what their needs are, facing the negative as well as the positive, judging oneself, establishing ties, needing to know what one is looking for, and truly caring for someone or something. These insights would seem to relate to leadership in terms of leader-follower relationships, the significance of goals, the need to be creative, and the importance of self-knowledge, passion and commitment.

Poetry

The poem "If" by Rudyard Kipling (1936, pp. 65–66) could be used in a discussion of leadership and the process of becoming a leader. In this familiar work, a father speaks to his son as the boy grows to manhood. The father tells the son to trust himself even when others doubt him, not to lie or hate others, to dream, to take risks, to retain his humanity and humility, and to "hold on when there's nothing in you except the will that says to [others] 'hold on.'" Students might be asked to compare the qualities this father ascribes to "a man" to those needed for effective leadership. Future discussion could center on the qualities that might be ascribed to "a woman," how they relate to leaders, and how women and men might lead differently.

Robert Frost's poem, "The Road Not Taken," (1949, p. 131) also can be used to stimulate students to reflect on the process of decision making. In the poem, the traveler makes the difficult decision to choose the path that is less worn and, for him, "that has made all the difference." Nursing students might be asked to consider the kinds of decisions leaders need to make if they are to articulate a vision, empower others, facilitate change, and manage conflict. They also could be asked to discuss the challenge of needing to make an unpopular decision—that is, choose the less-traveled path—and how they might approach such a situation.

Poetry and prose also have been used by Autry (1991) to illustrate and expand his perspectives on successful management, and by Cox (1994) to communicate her perspectives on nursing leadership and management. The poems included in Autry's text and Cox's article are ones written by the authors, rather than taken from elsewhere, and this provides a novel approach for nurse educators. In an attempt to determine if students are able to distinguish leadership from management, faculty might ask students to write a poem, a short story, or some other narrative form about each. Through this creative approach, faculty would be able to evaluate if students have learned and internalized the material rather than evaluating their ability to regurgitate the ideas of others, as happens so often in the traditional term paper format.

Film and Television

The 1979 film, *Norma Rae*, focuses on a poorly educated, underpaid, overworked factory worker who forges an alliance with a union worker and realizes the importance of solidarity and a common purpose. Despite threats and intimidations, Norma Rae (played by Sally Field in an Oscar-winning role) convinces her fellow workers that they can achieve better working conditions if they are willing to take a risk. The film ends with Norma Rae and a colleague organizing a union in her factory, rallying the workers to strike, and forcing management to negotiate with them. Certainly, this film could be used as a stimulus for a discussion of collective bargaining, unionization, and the ethical issues associated with strikes, particularly in health care or other service industries. But on a more general level, it also could be used to illustrate the leadership concepts of passion about and commitment to a goal, risk taking, the importance of leader-follower relationships, and the need for a leader to engage in self-reflection.

A more recent film, *Schindler's List* (1993), also depicts risk taking on the part of Oskar Schindler and the accountant who worked closely with him. Schindler's interest in the Jews of Poland began as a self-centered undertaking, where he hoped to employ cheap labor to make products that he could sell, thereby becoming a wealthy man. However, as he came to know his "employees" and understand their horrible plight, his goal became their safety and well-being. He took innumerable risks on behalf of "his Jews," lost vast sums of money, and changed his passions in life from "wine, women, and song" to compassion for his fellow human beings who were being grossly mistreated. Students of nursing might learn a great deal from Oskar Schindler's leadership and advocacy on behalf of the less fortunate, the underrepresented, the underserved. They might then use that understanding to suggest how they—as professional nurses caring for the homeless, the uninsured, and the alienated in our society—may need to serve as leaders to insure that all those who need care receive it.

The abuse of power is illustrated in the film, *Wall Street* (1987). In this film, Michael Douglas plays a Wall Street executive who will do anything to anybody in order to "come out on top." Initially he has a great deal of success, but eventually he fails in his relationships with others; people realize he is more interested in his own advancement than in them or anything else, and he fails. Although this executive is in a position of power and authority and seems to be successful initially, an analysis of his role over time might present students with some interesting "food for thought" about leaders and power.

The 1994 Disney film, *The Lion King*, provides excellent examples of how a position of authority does not automatically make one a true leader and how leaders can be swept up in their own grandness and potentially abuse their power. It also helps the viewer think about how an entire community could be helped to be whole and functional through the work of an effective leader. In this film, Simba, the young lion cub, cannot wait to be king so that he can tell everyone what to do and have no responsibilities; at least, that is his idea of what it means to be king. His evil uncle, Scar, plots to kill his brother and Simba so that he can inherit the throne, but Simba escapes. He spends many years in a distant land, in the company of some fun-loving friends, and gives up all hope of ever going home or being king. He finally realizes his responsibility to his community and returns to Pride Rock, knowing what he must do to restore the chaos, destruction, and lassitude that has evolved under Scar's rule. This wonderful story can be used in a study of leadership by asking students to analyze the leadership style of Mufasa and Scar and the effect of their styles on followers and the community at large, and then comparing their analyses with what they have found in the literature about leader effectiveness and leader–follower interdependence. They also could be asked to examine the growth of the young lion cub,

Simba, into the role of king and consider how that relates to their own growth as leaders.

Another Disney classic, *Fantasia* (1940), also may have some relevance to the study of leadership. In this story—which is supported by outstanding music—the apprentice to the local sorcerer commands a broom to carry water from the well outside to a container in the cabin. At first, he is pleased with his power and sits back lazily while the broom does his chore; soon, however, the broom splits and splits again until there are many brooms carrying water and the container in the cabin is overflowing. At this point, the apprentice does not know how to stop the madness and has lost control. This film provides the opportunity to reflect on the knowledge base needed if one is to exercise leadership, the difference between leading and "dumping a task" onto others, the need for leaders to be intimately involved in all aspects of an activity rather than sitting idly by while others do the work, and the need to know one's limitations as well as strengths when providing leadership.

The popular television program, *MASH* also could be used in a study of leadership. Although this series is no longer aired in prime time, it is available on videotape and on syndicated channels; thus, it is still a viable choice. Many of the characters in this award-winning program display leadership in various episodes. Over the years this show was produced, Margaret Hoolihan, the chief nurse, evolved from a quiet, docile person to a woman who knew what she wanted "her nurses" to be, asserted herself, took charge when necessary, and provided leadership within her scope of responsibility and within the *MASH* unit as a whole. Her character could be analyzed in terms of her leadership abilities, as well as the challenges a woman faces when attempting to provide leadership in a male-dominated system. Hawkeye Pierce also was able to mobilize others to act, held strong convictions about the care of the wounded, and would not ask others to do anything he would not do himself. These are but two examples of characters in this show who could be used in the study of leadership.

Television also provides the opportunity to examine the lives of significant people in history. The Biography series on a cable channel brings to life the struggles, values, visions, and actions of many well-known individuals, and it can be used to help students learn about what it means to be a leader and how one develops or evolves as a leader.

Fine Arts

Drama

The very popular play, *Les Misérables* (1987), tells the story of a man who escapes from prison after serving 19 years; he had stolen a loaf of bread to feed his sister's starving child. Upon being befriended by a priest soon after his release, the main character vows to change his name, change his location, and start a new life, which he does. He eventually comes to assume responsibility for and raise the daughter of a former employee of his who died. In the midst of this personal struggle, however, 18th century France is caught in the upheaval of revolution, and the main character becomes involved in that fight. *Les Misérables* is a story of needing to be oneself, being true to one's values, and being a part of a larger effort. The young students who attempt to organize the peasants to rise up against the tyranny of the elite class provide an example of individuals with a vision of a freer France, efforts to mobilize the masses or the potential followers in their cause, and failure in those efforts. The song "Do You Hear the People Sing?" challenges the masses to join in the crusade, be strong and stand with the students/leaders, refuse to be put down and ignored, and strive toward their dreams. The entire play, or this song in particular, could be used to analyze the strategies used to motivate people, leader/follower relationships, ways to convey a vision, and the reality of personal struggle in attempting to make change. As such, it would seem to have relevance in the study of the concept of leadership.

Another play, *West Side Story* (1957), also might be used to help students learn about leadership. This story of two New York City gangs with different values and cultural norms illustrates many sources of conflict and the resolution of conflict through violence. It can be used to stimulate a discussion of sources of conflict, how to deal with conflict, how to move toward change when the norms of a system are well entrenched, and how different characters in each gang provided leadership to the group.

Music

As noted earlier, if one is to be a leader, one must have a vision about a better tomorrow. Using the idea behind the song, "If I

Ruled the World," sung by Tony Bennett, students could be asked to complete the verses of that song in a way that reflects their visions for the future, visions of the world, their communities, or the nursing profession. Students' visions could then be compared, similarities noted and differences discussed, and formulation of specific strategies needed to realize those visions could be undertaken. Such an exercise challenges students to think about and articulate their ideas of a better world and then contemplate what they would need to do, personally and in collaboration with others, to turn those dreams into reality.

Stimulating students to think about a leader's responsibility for shaping a desirable future can also occur through the use of the song, "In the Year 2525" by Zager and Evans. This is a song about what the world may look like in the future: artificial insemination as the norm, picking babies from the bottom of a long glass tube, environmental destruction, and the demise of the entire world. Without a doubt, this song paints a bleak picture of the future. Despite the bleakness however, the possible reality described in this song could be used to initiate an analysis of the trends occurring in nursing practice and health care, the desirability of those trends, whether there is a way to change those trends, how trends start in the first place, and how to create a preferred future, rather than merely settling for what is likely to occur. Students could then be challenged to think of themselves as change agents and leaders, identify a trend they would like to reverse, and suggest things they could realistically do to work toward that end.

Contemporary music also could be used to stimulate self reflection. Michael Jackson's "Man in the Mirror" makes listeners think about their own responsibility in making change. As each of us looks in the mirror, we must be able to live with the person we see and be satisfied that we have done all we can do. Leaders also must be confident enough in their visions and their fellow followers that they can look in the mirror with pride and take responsibility for making needed changes.

Barbra Streisand's "Everybody Says Don't" tells about one individual's reactions to everybody saying "don't." This song tells us to walk on the grass, tilt at the windmill, make a noise, try, make a ripple, be brave, and don't be afraid. It inspires us and challenges us to take risks because at one point in time we may cause only a ripple, but the next time we could cause a wave. It could be used as a framework for students to think of themselves and their nursing colleagues as independent thinkers, risk takers, and change agents. It should be remembered, however, that Streisand's song has a very fast pace and without the words, it is difficult to discern the message; therefore, it is recommended that, if this song were to be used, the words be distributed to students before the song is played so they are not frustrated by an inability to understand all the words.

As noted in the discussion of leadership, leaders are change agents. They envision new orders or goals, and they motivate and mobilize others to work together to create that change. But change does not always happen in a planned, systematic way. Students can be assisted to reflect on the nature of change and how to manage it by listening to the words of two songs, "The Times They Are a Changin'" by Bob Dylan and "Revolution" by the Beatles. The former song suggests evolutionary change, where new practices, new standards, and new expectations seem to arise out of nowhere. The latter song, in contrast, acknowledges that not everyone is satisfied with such slow, albeit dramatic, change; instead, some people prefer a quicker, revolutionary approach to change. A discussion of the advantages and disadvantages of each type of change, the role of and demands on leaders and followers in each approach, and our experiences with each type in nursing's history may help students contemplate the changes needed in our society and our profession, as well as the most effective ways to affect them.

Finally, the music of the group, Sweet Honey in the Rock, and the story behind the group itself could be used in discussions of leadership. Sweet Honey in the Rock is an a capella group consisting of six African American women, started in 1973 by Bernice Johnson Reagon, a member of the group since its inception. Ms. Reagon wanted to find some way to make people be more aware of the richness of the African American culture, create a community of people, and bring people together with greater understanding. Having this vision led her to create Sweet Honey in the Rock and maintain it as a group that performs in local communities and for large groups throughout the world. The music of this group stimulates the listener to think about the spirit of community, social injustice, peace and justice issues, the strengths that each of us has, and cultural similarities and differences (Sweet Honey in the Rock, 1993, 1995); but it also serves as an excellent example of how one woman has served as a leader in mobilizing many people to be concerned about their fellow human beings. Sweet Honey in the Rock—its music and its history—can be a valuable resource in the study of leaders and leadership.

Painting

One very moving painting by Eugene Delacroix is entitled "Liberty Leading the People." This painting depicts a woman, tattered from being in battle and raising a flag above the rubble of the battlefield in an effort to lead the people in their continued fight. Looking at this scene may stimulate students to ask questions about and discuss the role of women in providing leadership, the losses one often suffers or the barriers that often need to be scaled before one's vision become a reality, how to keep followers motivated in moving toward a goal when all hope seems lost, or the kind of support leaders need as they fulfill that very challenging role. All of these areas are appropriate if we are to help students truly understand the complex phenomenon known as leadership.

Another painting of a woman who conveys some element of leadership is "The Madonna of Mercy" by Piero della Francesca. The madonna is shown to be a huge figure in comparison to the other people in the painting. She is standing with her arms extended wide and shielding a number of people under her cape. Her expression is one of caring and compassion, and that on the faces of those being watched over is one of adoration and gratitude. Students might be asked to study this work of art and think about the tasks of leadership as formulated by Gardner (1989, 1990), considering such questions as the following: What is the madonna doing to achieve a workable unity with this group of individuals? How is she serving as a symbol for them? What might you expect her to do were she to represent the group to external constituencies? How might her actions serve to renew members of the group? Even though this is not a moving figure whose words, actions, and thoughts are known, students can still make some assumptions about her role as a leader and her relationship to the group of followers depicted. They then could be asked to reflect on the assumptions they have made and how making assumptions might positively or negatively influence the effectiveness of a leader.

Additionally, Barratt's painting of "Florence Nightingale Receiving the Wounded at Scutari" portrays leadership. In this scene, wave after wave of wounded are being brought to the field hospital where Nightingale receives them with compassion. But lest one think Nightingale will do little more than hold the hands of the wounded, one sees in her expression the sense of control, the determination, and the quiet courage that was needed to improve the care of these soldiers and reverse the horrendous morbidity and mortality rates that existed. Students might be asked to view this painting on their own, list the characteristics of a leader evident in it, reflect on the significant role Nightingale played in changing battlefield care of the wounded, and examine "the founder of modern nursing" in terms of her leadership. Although students can and will read about Nightingale's accomplishments, a painting such as this seems to bring the woman to life and portray her as a real human being—which is what leaders are—not just some idealized heroine.

Sculpture

There are many pieces of sculpture that seem to portray power and leadership. "The Standing Woman" by LaChaise (previously described) presents a powerful, dominant figure who conveys confidence and a positive sense of self. Likewise, Michelangelo's "David" and contemporary sculptures of Abraham Lincoln, John F. Kennedy, George Washington, and Josef Stalin all are realistic portrayals of powerful people who surely had an effect on the world. In viewing such pieces, students might be challenged to consider how powerful men and women have been immortalized in society, how they would like to be portrayed were a sculpture to be cast of them, and what kind of sculpture they think would adequately and accurately convey the essence of leadership in nursing in today's world and the world of tomorrow.

CONCLUSION

It is evident from this discussion that leadership is a complex phenomenon and that learning about leadership and learning to be an effective leader are no easy tasks. The intricacies of leadership and how it differs from management, however, can be ascertained from various art forms, including poetry, children's stories and fables, novels, films, and historical works. These, combined with the multitude of books and articles about the topic could make the study of this very important concept enjoyable and informative for nursing students.

REFERENCES

Adams, R. (1972). *Watership down.* New York: Avon Books.

Ansbro, J. J. (1982). *Martin Luther King, Jr.: The making of a mind.* Maryknoll, NY: Orbis Books.

Autry, J. A. (1991). *Love and profit.* New York: William Morrow & Co.

Barnum, B. (1987). The need for heros and the need for brave men. *Courier, 54*(1), 5.

Bass, B. M. (1990). *Bass and Stodgill's handbook of leadership: Theory, research and managerial applications* (3rd ed.). New York: Free Press.

Bennis, W. G. (1989a). *On becoming a leader.* Reading, MA: Addison–Wesley.

Bennis, W. G. (1989b). Where have all the leaders gone? In W. E. Rosenbach & R. L. Taylor (Eds.), *Contemporary issues in leadership* (2nd ed., pp. 5–23). Boulder, CO: Westview Press.

Bennis, W., & Nanus, B. (1985). *Leaders: The strategies for taking charge.* New York: Harper & Row.

Brown, B. (1980). Follow the leader. *Nursing Outlook, 28*(6), 357–359.

Burns, J. M. (1978). *Leadership.* New York: Harper Torchbooks.

Corona, D. F. (1986). Followership: The indispensable corollary to leadership. In E. C. Hein & M. J. Nicholson (Eds.), *Contemporary leadership behavior: Selected readings* (2nd ed., pp. 87–91). Boston: Little, Brown.

Cox, M. (1994). Poetry in leadership: An enhancer of relationships. *Nursing Forum, 29*(1), 30–34.

DePree, M. (1989). *Leadership is an art.* New York: Dell.

de Saint-Exupéry, A. (1943). *The little prince.* New York: Harcourt Brace Jovanovich.

DiRienzo, S. M. (1994). A challenge to nursing: Promoting followers as well as leaders. *Holistic Nursing Practice, 9*(1), 26–30.

Frost, R. (1949). *Complete poems of Robert Frost.* New York: Henry Holt & Co.

Gardner, J. W. (1989). The tasks of leadership. In W. E. Rosenbach & R. L. Taylor (Eds.), *Contemporary issues in leadership* (2nd ed., pp. 24–33). Boulder, CO: Westview Press.

Gardner, J. W. (1990). *On leadership.* New York: The Free Press.

Gardner, J. W. (1993). The antileadership vaccine. In W. E. Rosenbach & R. L. Taylor (Eds.), *Contemporary issues in leadership* (3rd ed., pp. 193–200). Boulder, CO: Westview Press.

Goodwin, D. K. (1994). *No ordinary time. Franklin and Eleanor Roosevelt: The home front in World War II.* New York: Simon & Schuster.

Guidera, M. K., & Gilmore, C. (1988). In defense of followership. *American Journal of Nursing, 88*(7), 1017.

Kelley, R. E. (1989). In praise of followers. In W. E. Rosenbach & R. L. Taylor (Eds.), *Contemporary issues in leadership* (2nd ed., pp. 124–134). Boulder, CO: Westview Press.

Kelley, R. E. (1992). *The power of followership: How to create leaders people want to follow and followers who lead themselves.* New York: Doubleday Currency.

Kipling, R. (1936). "If." In H. Felleman (Selected by), *The best loved poems of the American people* (pp. 65–66). Garden City, NY: Doubleday & Co.

Lee, C. (1993). Followership: The essence of leadership. In W. E. Rosenbach & R. L. Taylor (Eds.), *Contemporary issues in leadership* (3rd ed., pp. 113–121). Boulder, CO: Westview Press.

Ludlum, R. (1988). *The icarus agenda.* New York: Random House.

Machiavelli, N. (1966). *The prince.* New York: Bantam Books.

Malone, B. (1990, April). The dawn of a new decade: Empowerment of nurses by nurses. Paper presented at the MSN Convention, Orlando, FL.

Manfredi, C. M., & Valiga, T. M. (1990). How are we preparing nurse leaders?: A study of baccalaureate curricula. *Journal of Nursing Education, 29*(1), 4–9.

Mitchell, S. (1988). *Tao te ching* (A new English version). New York: HarperPerennial.

Moloney, M. M. (1979). *Leadership in nursing: Theory, strategies, action.* St. Louis: Mosby.

Naisbitt, J., & Aburdene, P. (1990). *Megatrends 2000: Ten new directions for the 1990's.* New York: William Morrow & Co.

Piper, W. (1961). *The little engine that could.* New York: Platt & Munk.

Rost, J. (1985, October). Distinguishing leadership and management: A new consensus. Paper presented at the Organizational Development Network National Conference, San Francisco, CA.

Rost, J. C. (1994). Leadership: A new conception. *Holistic Nursing Practice, 9*(1), 1–8.

Silverstein, S. (1974). "The little blue engine." In S. Silverstein, *Where the sidewalk ends* (p. 158). New York: Harper and Row.

Sweet Honey in the Rock. (1993). *Still on the journey* (insert booklet with compact disc). Redway, CA: EarthBeat! Records.

Sweet Honey in the Rock. (1995). *NLN Update, 1*(1), 2.

VanFleet, D. D., & Yukl, G. A. (1989). A century of leadership research. In W. E. Rosenbach & R. L. Taylor (Eds.), *Contemporary issues in leadership* (2nd ed., pp. 65–94). Boulder, CO: Westview Press.

Williams, M. (1975). *The velveteen rabbit*. New York: Avon Books.

Zaleznik, A. (1977). Managers and leaders: Are they different? *Harvard Business Review, 55*(3), 67–78.

14

Professionalism

One of the purposes of a nursing education program is to socialize students into the role of the professional nurse. Students need to learn about the values that are congruent with professional practice, integrate those values into their own daily practice, gain insights about the image they convey, learn about the public's image of nurses and nursing, and function in a responsible, professional manner. Achieving such goals, however, is no small task, nor does it occur overnight.

Unlike many other concepts that are integral to a nursing education, learning about professionalism and learning to be a professional are pervasive throughout the educational experience. In a curriculum, the material on assessment, for example, may be limited to a single course. The same may be true for content related to family systems, wellness, or leadership. But learning about professionalism begins with a student's first day in the program—and possibly even before that—and continues until graduation and beyond.

Thinking of one's self as a responsible professional nurse rather than a student, a mother, a worker in another field, or someone merely out to enjoy life and have a good time, can be a difficult transition for many students. In addition, students are confronted with the challenge of thinking of themselves as investigators, health teachers, advocates, members of interdisciplinary teams, and change agents who practice in any number of acute, long-term, or community-based settings. This compounds the difficulties inherent in learning professionalism.

Nurse educators need to be aware of the multiple dimensions of the concept of professionalism and be sensitive to the challenges that accompany helping students take on the responsibilities associated with a professional nursing role. It also is necessary to consider how students can be helped to learn about professionalism and incorporate professional characteristics into their own value systems.

The elements of professionalism are many, but the focus for this discussion will center on the following: values and ethics, collaboration, one's personal strengths and weaknesses, and image. In addition, examples of how the arts and humanities can facilitate learning about the concept of professionalism will be offered.

ELEMENTS OF PROFESSIONALISM

Values and Ethics

The nursing profession has struggled for years with the question of whether nursing is a profession or an occupation, and this is a debate about which students need to be aware. Perhaps the most commonly used criteria for determining whether a group is a profession or not are those proposed by Abraham Flexner in 1915. Flexner's criteria have been modified by subsequent authors, and the following have evolved as typical criteria used:

1. the activities of members of the group are based on a body of knowledge that has been developed through research and theory testing;
2. the body of knowledge is unique;
3. the body of knowledge can be learned, and it is usually acquired through a long period of study, in a specified "curriculum," taught by members of the group itself;
4. members of the group have some internal organization through which they address relevant issues and concerns;
5. members of the group share a common identity and purpose;
6. members of the group are guided by a code of ethics;
7. members of the group regulate their own education and practice through peer review and other mechanisms; and
8. members of the group are motivated by altruism or a desire to provide for the good of society; they are oriented toward service rather than personal gain.

Perhaps the most significant questions which nurse educators must help students address, are not whether nursing is a profession or what the barriers are that may keep it from becoming a full profession. Instead, the most significant questions are what makes a group come to be acknowledged as a profession by society, what do members of that group do that leads them to be viewed as professionals, and what do nurses and nursing need to do to be recognized as a well-established, highly regarded profession and to maintain that status.

Questions such as these relate more to the values inherent in nurses' practice and their interactions with patients and families than do to the number of nurses who are members of the American Nurses Association, for example. It is those values that educators must clarify for and transmit to students, and it is those values that students need to internalize. But what are the values that characterize professional nursing practice?

Among the tenets that guide professional nursing practice are those of *holism and individualistic care*. Perhaps more than any other health care providers, nurses concern themselves with the psychosocial and spiritual dimension of the patient, not only with the physical dimension. Nurses attend to the meaning that an illness has for a patient and his family, and not only to the illness itself as may be the focus of a physician. Likewise, nurses do not concentrate only on the spiritual needs of the individual, as may be true for a pastoral counselor; instead, nurses also are concerned with the needs of the individual's physical condition, his family, and so on. In addition, when nurses plan care, they attend to the individual needs of the patient, and they intervene in personalized, individualized ways. Thus, the notions of holism and individualized care are integral to professional nursing practice, and students must learn how to practice in ways that reflect these values.

The practice of professional nursing also reflects the value of *integrity*. Included in this dimension of practice are the ideas of confidentiality and protecting the patient's right to privacy; nurses hold in confidence information given to them by or gathered about patients, and they share pertinent information only with appropriate members of the health care team. Integrity also includes assuming responsibility and accountability for patient care outcomes; nurses practice within the scope of designated legal parameters, and they take responsibility for the care provided within that scope of practice. In addition, nurses are expected to be trustworthy, reliable, dependable, and honest. It is expected that, as they engage in their various roles, professional nurses will act to protect patients from harm, involve them in decision making, recognize and respect their rights, treat them with dignity and respect, and be guided by the *Code for Nurses* (American Nurses Association, 1976), the profession's ethical code of conduct. Finally, they are expected to report unethical or abusive behavior exhibited by any member of the health care team. All of these behaviors reflect the notion of personal integrity.

Professional nursing practice also reflects the valuing of *autonomy*. Nurses who engage in professional practice have control over their own practice and are not handmaidens or subservient to other health professionals. Autonomous practice requires a certain degree of self-confidence in one's abilities, clarity regarding one's scope of practice, assertiveness, and willingness to make decisions and accept responsibility for consequences.

Without a doubt, the practice of professional nursing values *caring*. The relationships that nurses form with patients are based on a genuine concern for the patient's well-being, and that attitude of concern is reflected in the nurse's actions. Additionally, a caring relationship is reciprocal, where both the nurse and the patient give of themselves and both benefit from the mutual concern. Thus, the element of caring is integral to the practice of professional nursing and is a value that students must integrate into their educational experience and their careers.

Nursing also values the concept of *advocacy*. As an advocate for patients, families, and nursing, professional nurses are called upon to speak for others who are unable or unwilling to speak for themselves. The goal of assuming the role of advocate is to ensure that all individuals are treated fairly, competently, and with respect, to promote patient autonomy, to protect patients' rights, and to see that patient preferences are integral to any decisions that are made. In today's fast-paced, impersonal, ever-changing health care environment, the nurse's role as advocate is becoming increasingly important, and nursing students will need to develop great skill in this aspect of professionalism.

Among the values significant to the nursing profession is that of *competence*. It is expected that professional nurses are knowledgeable and skilled and that their competence is used to the benefit of patients and their families. As they care for, teach, counsel, advocate for, and communicate with the recipients of care, professional nurses demonstrate that nursing practice is based on knowledge, that nurses think critically, and that the skills performed by them are done at an expert level. Professional nurses maintain their competence by *engaging in ongoing education* and by maintaining *active involvement in professional associations*, two additional elements of professionalism about which students must learn.

Finally, the nursing profession values having a *career focus*, not merely a job orientation. Professional nurses, as students come to learn, see themselves as investing in the future of the profession itself. They take responsibility for the health of the profession, work to promote nursing's visibility, acknowledge the accomplishments of those in the field, publish, engage in research, share ideas with lay and professional groups, and take responsibility for the development of the profession's new members. Professionalism incorporates a long-term, far-reaching investment in the profession, rather than a narrow, self-centered, short-term perspective.

Collaboration

In addition to these internal values, professionalism involves working collaboratively with other health care providers. This collaboration will become increasingly important as health care becomes more complex, delivery systems become integrated, and knowledge and specialization continue to explode. Indeed, "in the future it is likely that health care delivery will be provided by groups of health professionals utilizing a team approach" (Moloney, 1992, p. 233).

In essence, "the delivery of health care to patients involves a number of professionals and paraprofessionals in complex, interactive, collaborative relationships" (Hinshaw, 1990, p. 17), and students of nursing need to become skilled in these kinds of relationships. Collaboration means mutually working together to define and reach goals. It incorporates cooperation, but is more than that. It involves mutuality, trust, mutual respect, sharing information, feeling secure about oneself and one's role, recognizing the worth of self and others, encouraging creativity in others, and being supportive of others.

In essence, collaboration involves interdependence, giving help without being overly powerful, and accepting help without feeling powerless. In order to be interdependent with others, professional nurses need to know what their expertise is, to be clear about what it is that they have to offer, and not to feel threatened by working with others. Nursing students need to be helped to clarify just what it is that makes a nurse a nurse . . . what it is that is unique about nursing and what nurses have to offer . . . and what it is that distinguishes nurses from other health care providers, such as physicians, and from other caregivers, such as mothers. Answering such questions is no easy task.

According to Moloney (1992, p. 233), "efforts at collaboration are rather difficult for many nurses because they have not been socialized for such roles early in their preparation." If this claim has merit, nursing students need to be exposed to and participate in learning experiences that put them in contact with other health care professionals, help them learn about the roles of others, challenge them to appreciate the team approach to care, and help them understand the unique contributions of everyone involved in providing complex care to patients and their families. Faculty are challenged, therefore, to design learning experiences that would achieve these goals.

Personal Strengths and Weaknesses

One of the hallmarks of professionals is that they have a degree of expertise in a given area, and those with less knowledge in that area look to them for advice and counsel. Professionals also are competent and skilled at what they do.

Despite this expertness, professionals also are well aware of how much there is yet to learn, realize that knowledge is ever-changing, and acknowledge that they must continually learn new skills and continue their education in formal or informal ways. How they decide where to focus their energies, however, is based on a careful analysis of their own strengths and limitations.

One important element of the concept of professionalism, therefore, is being aware of one's strengths or talents, being clear about the areas that need further development if one is to practice at a high level of competence and expertise, and choosing to engage in activities that will build upon those strengths and overcome limitations. In essence, self-assessment is a crucial aspect of professionalism that must be initiated early in one's career. Thus, students in nursing programs need to learn about their own strengths and weaknesses and how to deal with them.

If nursing students are to develop as professionals, educators must expose them to learning experiences that will "force" them to examine what they know and do not know, what their values are, how their behaviors are influenced by their values, what they can do well and what they need to improve, and what strategies they can pursue to help them become more effective professionals. It is only with this kind of honest, critical self-appraisal that students will be prepared to practice in a professional way and contribute effectively to the health care team.

NURSING'S IMAGE

It is no secret that "nursing is simply not perceived as a high-status, powerful health profession" (Andreoli, Carollo, & Pottage, 1990, p. 41). Despite the extraordinary gains made by members of the nursing profession over the years, our image "continues to be a major problem for the profession today" (Porter, Porter, & Lower, 1990, p. 51). Nurse educators need to acknowledge this with students, but they also need to help students understand the complexities of this issue so that strategies to improve nursing's image can be instituted.

As noted in the literature (Paul, 1991; Porter, et al., 1990; Roberts, 1983; Stafford, 1987; Yura, 1989), many things affect the image of nurses and nursing. Among them are the opinions nurses hold of themselves, including whether or not they experience a sense of powerlessness, low self-esteem, self-hatred (Roberts, 1983), or submissiveness. Nursing's image also is tarnished through "horizontal violence" (Fanon as cited in Roberts, 1983, p. 23), where nurses fail to support each other rather than working actively to promote their nursing colleagues. Additionally, nurses' lack of political action also contributes to a less-than-positive image, and the failure to publicize what they do and how that makes a difference in people's lives (Chandler, 1992) keeps nursing from enjoying the kind of image it deserves.

In essence, "a clear, positive image of professional nursing . . . depends on what nurses understand about themselves and how well they convey that understanding to others" (Hein & Nicholson, 1990, p. 1). Strasen (1992) goes so far as to assert that "effective and lasting changes for the image of professional nursing must focus on changing the self-image of each individual nurse" (p.viii).

She outlines a self-image model (see Figure 14.1) that integrates the individual's thoughts and beliefs about self, self-image, actions, and public image, and she suggests that there needs to be more attention paid to the self-image individual nurses hold of themselves.

Figure 14.1 Self-Image Model *

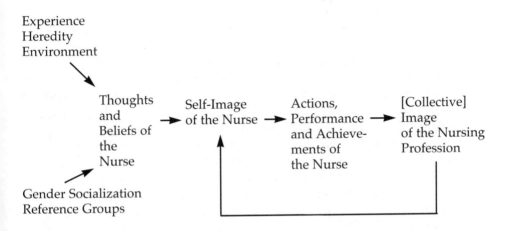

* Source: Strasen, L. L. (1992). *The image of professional nursing: Strategies for action* (p. viii & p. 31). Philadelphia: Lippincott. Reprinted with permission.

The image of nurses, therefore, involves knowing and believing in self, knowing and living up to one's potential, and being able to truly "see" oneself (Bennis, 1989; Brower, 1983). It also involves the ways in which nurses express themselves verbally and in writing, their actions, and the way they present themselves, including how they dress.

Clothing is a form of nonverbal communication that reflects confidence in one's ability and judgment, personal behavior, and sense of professionalism. Curtin (1985) insists, therefore, that nurses should dress, not so much for success—as the titles of many books and articles would have us believe—but for respect.

Image also involves personal integrity. By personal integrity is meant the ability to make and keep commitments to ourselves and to others, to "walk our talk," and to have honor with ourselves (Covey, 1989). In a word, personal integrity means authenticity.

The literature in nursing and other fields offers numerous strategies to change and improve the image of nursing. Kalisch and Kalisch (1990) focused particularly on influencing how nurses are portrayed in the media. Andreoli et al. (1990) outlined a comprehensive marketing plan for improving the image of nursing, including acknowledging that nurses themselves must be considered a target audience. Porter et al. (1990) suggested that nurses improve their image by working as consultants, collaborating with physicians, increasing their scholarliness, increasing their involvement in professional organizations, and empowering one another. And Strasen (1992), working on the assumptions basic to the self-image model she outlined, suggested that nursing's image will be improved when nurses set clear goals for themselves, work actively to meet those goals, assume total responsibility for themselves, engage in critical self-assessments, continue their education, and acknowledge their own and their nursing colleagues' accomplishments.

Why do we need to be concerned about image as a component of professionalism? Perhaps it is because "public opinion is vital to the success of social, political, and professional groups in attaining their goals" (Kalisch & Kalisch, 1990, p. 33). Public opinion, or the public image of nursing, also affects the number and quality of persons who are drawn to the profession, and it affects policymakers who make decisions regarding the allocation of resources. Finally, public opinion also affects nurses' self-image and self-confidence.

Thus, the educational process must attend to the image of the nurse in the past and at present. And students must be helped to be aware of the image they convey, assess whether that image is congruent with the one they want the public to have of the profession, and propose strategies to improve their own image and the image of the profession as a whole.

SUMMARY

The concept of professionalism is a multifaceted one that involves the values that characterize nursing practice, working collaboratively with a variety of health care professionals, being aware of one's personal strengths and weaknesses, and promoting a positive image. Students of nursing need to be helped to learn and incorporate the values that are significant for professional practice, develop the skills needed for effective collaboration, analyze their own abilities, and convey a positive image. Since many of these outcomes require introspection, reflection, and personal analysis, learning experiences that bring students in contact with ethical dilemmas, varying images of the nurse, positive and negative nurse-physician relationships, and opportunities for self-evaluation are needed. The arts and humanities can provide some of these types of learning experiences.

THE ARTS AND HUMANITIES RELATED TO PROFESSIONALISM

Following are a number of examples of works from the arts and humanities that can be used to help nursing students learn about the concept of professionalism and internalize professional values. However, two resources deserve particular attention since they offer numerous examples that could be used in nursing education.

Images of Nurses: Perspectives from History, Art, and Literature, edited by Anne Hudson Jones (1988), presents examples of the images of nurses that have been portrayed since pre-Nightingale times. This book discusses the image of nursing portrayed in a 1936 Hollywood film about Florence Nightingale, as well as in several pieces of literature, including novels, poems, and short stories. In addition, it includes numerous examples from the fine arts, including sculpture, architecture, paintings, carved cabinets, and photographs, that depict nurses and the work of nurses. The photographs included in the book are all black and white, which detracts from their richness to some extent, but they nevertheless offer a range of views of nurses and nursing and could be used in nursing education.

M. Patricia Donahue's *Nursing: The Finest Art* (1985) presents an illustrated history of the profession as evidenced in paintings, photographs, stamps, sculpture, sketches, and recruitment posters. This beautiful full-color book depicts how the role of the nurse has changed over the centuries, as well as how elements of nursing— such as compassion and caring—have remained intact despite societal and professional turmoil.

In addition to these two general resources that offer educators many works of art for use in their teaching, there are a number of specific examples of literature, film, paintings, sculpture, and so on that have relevance to the educational experiences of nursing students. Some of those specific examples are offered here for the reader's consideration.

Literature

Novels

Intensive Care: The Story of a Nurse (Heron, 1987) and *The Nurse's Story* (Gino, 1982) are realistic accounts of individual nurses in practice. Both books are easy to read, and both offer specific clinical situations as well as these nurses' responses to and roles in them. Other examples of similar books that may be used to help students learn about professional roles and values, collaboration with other members of the health care team, and the image of the nurse include *Children's Hospital* (Anderson, 1985), *The Nurses* (Frede, 1985), and *Delivery: A Nurse–Midwife's Story* (Crichton, 1986).

Children's Hospital (Anderson, 1985) is an account of the true story of six children and their families. Each of the children had been hospitalized in a specialized children's hospital in an urban area because of a serious and, for the most part, lengthy illness. The stories convey the frustrations experienced by the children, their parents, the nurses, and the physicians as all struggle with difficult situations and the possibility of death. But they also relay the kinds of relationships that can evolve between nurses and patients, the ways in which the nurses become intimately involved with their patients, the knowledge and skills needed by nurses as they face a variety of clinical challenges, and the roles of the nurses as advocates, teachers, leaders, and care givers. Although it makes for fascinating story telling, the six cases are not presented separately; instead, the story of each child is told throughout the book, which makes it difficult for faculty to assign a student to read and analyze the case of one child/family. Despite this limitation, however, the book offers thoughtful portrayals of professional nurses in practice.

In *The Nurses* (Frede, 1985), the physicians in this inner-city hospital go on strike, and the nurses stay on the units to deliver care. The story revolves around a nurse practitioner, a head nurse, and a group of nursing staff who are extraordinarily dedicated to their patients. Included among the nursing staff is a male whose wife left him because she felt he could not be a "real man" if he were a nurse. In addition to addressing the issue of health care workers striking and the ethics of that kind of action, this book could be used to focus on several other trends and issues in nursing: the role of nurse practitioners, the leadership style of the head nurse, nurse-physician relationships, the challenges to men in a primarily female profession, and the potential for "burnout" among staff.

Set in a hospital for inner-city poor patients, most of whom have high-risk pregnancies, *Delivery: A Nurse–Midwife's Story* (Crichton, 1986) tells about the role of a nurse midwife who is dedicated to natural childbirth. The story provides numerous clinical examples of high-risk pregnancies and difficult births; but it also depicts the professional, independent role of a nurse midwife and how she must "fight the odds" to help women through natural childbirths when "the system" tends to intervene to "move things along." It also includes a situation of a stillbirth, the impact of that experience on the nurse midwife as well as the parents, and how the nurse dealt with this very difficult situation. In assigning students to read this book, faculty might direct them to think about what it means to be an independent, autonomous professional, the challenges one often faces when trying to live one's values, how the nurse serves as an advocate for patients, how to manage conflicts with physicians and others, and how to function as an agent for change. *Delivery: A Nurse–Midwife's Story* offers numerous topics for discussion and can be used to meet many learning objectives.

In contrast to these true-to-life and serious accounts of the nurse working in the health care system, *The House of God* (Shem, 1978) is a humorous look at the inner life of a hospital. This book, written by a physician, focuses primarily on physicians and residents (interns) and the challenges they face; however, it also can be used to give nursing students an insight into the role of the physician so that they better appreciate the perspective of their health team colleagues in patient situations. In this novel one sees the many ways in which one's professional values can be challenged by the realities of a system that is life-and-death oriented, understaffed, and constantly changing. The book also depicts how care providers deal with stress, often in less-than-desirable ways. All of these situations are realities of today's health care system, making this book a viable stimulus for the analysis and discussion of several topics that relate to the concept of professionalism.

In addition to this fictitious account of professional practice that makes light of some serious clinical situations, faculty may want to consider using two other books that challenge nursing's usual ways of thinking and teaching: *The Sisterhood* (Palmer, 1982) and *Nurses Who Kill* (Linedecker & Burt, 1990). The former book is a work of fiction about a small group of nurses who engage in active euthanasia, the latter is a series of true accounts of the same phenomenon, but the "nurses" cited in these cases include aides and practical nurses as well as registered nurses. In both books, nurses are troubled by a system that strives to maintain life at all cost but seems to devalue the quality of life. Their solution is to "put the sufferers out of their misery" by killing them.

While it is true that the nursing profession does not promote active euthanasia, the ethical issues of suffering, prolonged dying, and unnecessary use of life-extending technology—issues that students need to discuss—are brought to light through these books, thereby making them useful in education. *The Sisterhood* and *Nurses Who Kill* can be used to explore the issues noted above and to stimulate discussions of values, caring for the terminally ill, the role of the professional nurse, whistle-blowing, how investigative skills and deductive thinking may lead one to suspect a fellow staff member of unethical behavior, and so on. These are difficult discussions, and reading these books is likely to be uncomfortable for students; therefore, it is suggested that they be used with students nearing completion of the program and that faculty give a sensitive introduction before assigning these readings. Faculty also must be clear about the purposes of assigning students to read these books, and be available to students if they become upset by the situations presented.

Students also might be challenged to think about the role of the nurse by reading excerpts from the mystery novel, *Shroud for a Nightingale* (James, 1971), which takes place in a hospital during the early part of the 20th century. At one point in the story, the following exchange takes place between two nurses:

> Every report and recommendation seems to take us further away from the bedside. We have dieticians to see to the feeding, physiotherapists to exercise the patients, [and so on]. . . . If we're not careful nursing will become a

residual skill, the job which is left when all the technicians have had their turn. . . . Ask yourself what is the function of the nurse today. What exactly are we trying to teach these girls?

. . . To obey orders implicitly and be loyal to their supervisors. Obedience and loyalty. Teach the students those and you've got a good nurse.

. . . That was good enough for our generation, but these kids ask whether the orders are reasonable before they start obeying and what their superiors have done to deserve their respect. A good thing too on the whole. How on earth do you expect to attract intelligent girls into nursing if you treat them like morons? We ought to encourage them to question established procedures, even to answer back occasionally. . . . Give me an intelligent girl and I'll make a good nurse of her whether she thinks she has a vocation or not. You can have the stupid ones. They may minister to your ego but they'll never make good professional women (P. D. James, 1971, pp. 137–138).

After reading this exchange, students could be asked to survey nurses in practice regarding the extent to which they value intelligence, obedience, questioning, and "answering back occasionally." They also might be asked to reflect on these things themselves. A lively discussion about the role of nurses, how their practice reflects their values, and what the basic values of professional nurses are could then follow.

The right-to-die issue and that of assisted suicide, both difficult ethical issues, are the focus of the book, *This Far and No More* (Malcolm, 1987). This is a true account of a determined, intelligent, accomplished, 40-year-old wife and mother who suffers from amyotrophic lateral sclerosis (ALS). It details her 3-year struggle with this debilitating disease, and tells of the emotional and financial burdens experienced by the central character and her family. Progressing from an active professional to a woman who is totally dependent on others for living, Emily Bauer experienced dramatic changes in all aspects of her life. The most difficult of these changes was the fact that "the mind, untouched, is sentenced to sit there inside the once-active person and witness the slow decay of its vibrant bodily shell, finger by finger, joint by joint, muscle by muscle, function by function, as if millions of ants were slowly crawling up the body sucking its vitality from within" (Malcolm, 1987, p. 38).

This very poignant, touching story—written in part by the dying woman herself and in part by her husband and friends—tells of her frustrations with her caregivers, her family, and the health care system; her anger, depression, and sense of helpless-ness; and her decision to take some degree of control of what was happening to her. Emily Bauer (a pseudonym) chose assisted sui-cide. *This Far and No More* could be used as a case study in which the role of the professional nurse is examined. How did the nurs-es in this story help Emily physically, emotionally, and spiritually? How did they help Emily's family? How does the health care sys-tem need to be altered to attend more to the needs and wishes of the patient? What is the role of an ethics committee in a situation like this? Are there situations in which nurses should participate in assisted suicides; if so, what are those situations? And so on.

This kind of a story clearly deals with decisions that need to be made by individuals. The novel, *Decisions* (Bright, 1984), also provides an opportunity for students to explore the nature of deci-sion making and consider their own decision making processes. This fictional account is about a woman who must make some dif-ficult decisions related to balancing her family responsibilities, her career demands, and her personal needs. Although the main char-acter in this book is an attorney, the dilemmas inherent in her situ-ation are similar to those experienced by many other professionals, including nurses. The book might be used most effectively, there-fore, with students nearing completion of a program as they con-template how they will "do it all" . . . pursue their professional careers, continue their education, establish families, become involved in their local communities and professional organiza-tions, and take time for themselves. Students could critique the decision making process used by the main character in this book, compare it with processes described in textbooks, and consider the clarity of their own processes.

Finally, the Charles Dickens (1910) classic, *Martin Chuzzlewit*, originally published in 1844, tells of mid-19th-century America and includes a character who is a nurse. Sairey Gamp, sadly, is a somewhat true representation of nurses before the reforms insti-tuted by Florence Nightingale. Sairey Gamp is large, slovenly, and frequently drunk; she neglects her patients and abuses them by punching them, strangling them, and placing them terribly close to open fires, all in the name of helping them; and she talks to anyone and everyone about her patients. Obviously, Mrs. Gamp is far from the ideal professional nurse, but this classic novel could be used to provide a yardstick against which to measure the behavior of nurs-es in practice. Students could be asked to consider questions such as, "What kind of image do nurses in your clinical area present to patients and other professionals?", "In what ways do nurses violate the privacy and confidentiality of patients, either consciously or unconsciously?", and "Are there subtle ways in which nurses 'abuse' patients?"

Short Stories and Children's Stories

A very poignant story that helps readers contemplate their values, goals, and relationships is the classic work, *Gift from the Sea* (Lindbergh, 1955). This is a story of a woman who takes a brief vacation by the sea. As she walks the shore and examines sea shells, she has the opportunity to think without being distracted by the details of everyday existence and to reflect on what is important to her in life. After reading this story, students might be directed to complete a self-assessment of their own values, strengths, abilities to relate to patients and other people, competencies, and weaknesses. They also might be required to outline a plan for ongoing personal and professional development that reflects the insights gained from the self-assessment, and include in that plan how they might continue that kind of self-analysis when they no longer have teachers and course assignments to "force" them to do it. Walking a quiet beach alone and paying attention to the "gifts from the sea," as Lindbergh did, might be a useful strategy for students to use themselves.

All I Really Need to Know I Learned in Kindergarten (Fulghum, 1986) is a simple, but thoughtful, reflection on values. In a light, humorous way, the author challenges the reader to think about basic values, like those learned in kindergarten—share everything, play fair, live a balanced life, be aware of wonder, and when you go out into the world, watch out for traffic, hold hands, and stick together. Students could be asked to read this short collection of thoughts and reflect on their own basic values. They also could be asked to debate the relevance of the "sandbox-type" values outlined in this book for professional nursing practice: Does "playing fair" have anything to do with honesty and professional integrity? Does "holding hands and sticking together" have anything to do with collegiality? Does "washing your hands before you eat" have anything to do with cleanliness? And does "remembering the most important word in the Dick-and-Jane books—LOOK" have anything to do with observational and assessment skills, problem identification, and being aware of one's surroundings?

A very useful children's story, *Hope for the Flowers* (Paulus, 1972), tells of a caterpillar who is dissatisfied with his life, "jumps on the bandwagon" to get to the top (even though he is not sure what is at the top!), and assumes a "climb or be climbed" (p. 25) attitude, based on the assumption that other caterpillars were threats and obstacles. But then he gets to know another caterpillar as an individual and finds that she is not a threat. The female caterpillar decides to give up the climb to the top, and encounters a wise worm who teaches her how to spin a cocoon so that she can be transformed into a butterfly. Although she is uncertain as to what may happen when she is inside a cocoon, she takes the risk and does become a beautiful butterfly. She then sets out to find her friend, who is still struggling to get to the top, and convinces him to spin a cocoon. She tells him, "You must want to fly so much that you are willing to give up being a caterpillar," (p. 75). Eventually, the two are able to soar above the crowds of caterpillars all climbing to the top and see that there is nothing at the top. This story conveys insights related to change, risk taking, realistic goal setting, decision making, mentoring, and realizing one's strengths and one's potentials. As such, it could serve as a focal point for a discussion of significant elements of the concept of professionalism.

Poetry

One of the greatest American poets, Walt Whitman, not only wrote about nurses, he himself was a volunteer nurse and companion to the wounded soldiers during the Civil War. His poem, "The Wound–Dresser" (Hollway, 1932, pp. lix–lx), is a moving account of the dedication needed and the challenges faced by nurses as they assume the role of caregiver. The following portion of this poem conveys the feelings and struggles experienced by Whitman, the nurse:

> I onward go, I stop,
> With hinged knees and steady hand to dress wounds,
> I am firm with each, the pangs are sharp yet unavoidable,
> One turns to me his appealing eyes—poor boy! I never knew you,
> Yet I think I could not refuse this moment to die for you, if that would
> > save you.

This poem could be used to initiate discussions about men in nursing, the intrapersonal conflicts that arise in nurses when they must perform painful treatments, the inner turmoil one experiences when wishing the suffering of another could be relieved but realizing it cannot be, and the times when one needs a "steady hand to dress wounds" even though those wounds may be purulent, gaping, and repulsive. Although the context in which Whitman wrote "The Wound–Dresser" is unlike that in which students practice, the challenges and dilemmas presented in this poem and the feelings it evokes could serve to stimulate self-reflection and evaluation, as well as a deeper understanding of what it means to be a professional nurse.

Florence Nightingale herself was the subject of poems written by Edward R. Campbell, Joyce Kilmer, Henry Wadsworth Longfellow, and Eleanor Ross Taylor, a contemporary poet. These poems reveal an image the public had of "the lady with the lamp," an image that told of the selfless, defiant, vigilant, ever-attentive nurse.

Campbell's "The Heroine of Scutari" (1857) tells how Nightingale defied the bureaucracy to obtain supplies needed for the wounded. Joyce Kilmer's "In Memoriam: Florence Nightingale" (1919), written at the time of her death, speaks of her compassion, gentle spirit, vanquishing of pain, and immortality, which referred to the lasting value of her work. "Santa Filomena", written in 1857 by Longfellow, was a tribute to Nightingale's goodness, heroic contributions, and attentiveness (Wagenknecht, 1986). And "Welcome Eumenides" by Eleanor Ross Taylor (1972) is a dramatic and powerful testament—using the words of Nightingale herself—to her strength, determination, personal sacrifice, and desire to strengthen the system of care for the wounded. Any or all of these poems could be used with nursing students to help them appreciate the profession's history, the personal characteristics of the founder of modern nursing, how the pubic image of nursing has or has not changed, and the personal strengths needed to deal with conflict and promote change, all of which are inherent in a study of professionalism in all its complexity.

A poem written for children, "This Bridge" (Silverstein, 1981), also has relevance for a study of professionalism. This poem tells of a bridge, provided by someone else, that will take the traveler to wondrous worlds his companion has known; however, in order to go places he himself would like to see, the traveler will have to take the last few steps alone. This short but meaningful poem can be used to challenge students to think about their own career directions, how they can use what others—teachers, textbooks, mentors, colleagues—can provide on that journey, and how they need to take responsibility for their own paths and directions. In talking about a career in nursing, students need to consider what it is they would like to do, the risks inherent in moving in new directions, and the support systems they have as they embark on such a journey; this poem can serve as the stimulus for such reflection and discussion.

"It Can Be Done" (Author Unknown, 1941) is a poem about stamina and positive thinking: ". . . We'd linger in the age of stone. The world would sleep if things were run by men who say, 'It can't be done'" (p. 274). And the need to take responsibility to act when there is a need for action is brought to light in the poem, "I Shall Not Pass this Way Again" (Felleman, 1936, p. 77):

Through this toilsome world, alas!
Once and only once I pass;
If a kindness I may show,
If a good deed I may do
To a suffering fellow man,
Let me do it while I can.
No delay, for it is plain
I shall not pass this way again.

Additionally, William Ernest Henley's "Invictus" (Felleman, 1936, p. 73)[1] inspires readers to reflect on the strengths they bring to the world and the control they can have in their lives:

Out of the night that covers me,
  Black as the Pit from pole to pole,
I thank whatever gods may be
  For my unconquerable soul.

In the fell clutch of circumstance
  I have not winced nor cried aloud.
Under the bludgeonings of chance
  My head is bloody, but unbowed.

---

1. Reprinted with the permission of Scribner, a Division of Simon & Schuster, from *Poems* by Willim Errest Henley (New York: Scribner, 1898).

Beyond this place of wrath and tears
        Looms but the Horror of the shade,
And yet the menace of the years
        Finds and shall find me unafraid.

It matters not how strait the gate,
        How charged with punishments the scroll,
I am the master of my fate:
        I am the captain of my soul.

The poem "Two Citadels" (Lindbergh, 1956, p. 9) could be used in a discussion of collegiality and collaboration. This poem tells of "two citadels of stone imprisoned in our worlds, two worlds that spin each in a separate orbit." But when they allow themselves to break out of those boundaries, they are able to enjoy life and accomplish so much more. Students could explore whether nurses and physicians have allowed themselves to become imprisoned in worlds that reflect traditional roles and stereotypes and, if so, how those walls could be broken down to allow for greater collaboration, which would benefit patients and families.

"The Road Not Taken" by Robert Frost, previously suggested for use in relation to the concept of leadership, also has relevance in a discussion of professionalism. This poem tells the story of a person who, upon walking in the woods, comes to a point where the road divides, and he must decide which path to take. He decides on the one that is less worn and less traveled. Students learning about what it means to be a professional might read this poem with an eye to contemplating the ethical dilemmas one often faces. They could read textbooks on ethical decision making, read this poem, interview nurses in practice about times when they have had to make difficult decisions and what the consequences of making the less "popular" decision were, and write an analysis of their own decision making processes when faced with a situation in their own clinical practice.

"Vashti" by Harper (1993) is a moving poem that brings to light the need to act in ways that are in accord with one's values. It tells of a queen who is summoned to her king to entertain his male companions. Vashti tells the messengers that before she would shame herself like that, she would take the crown from her head and die. Upon hearing this, the king banishes her from the kingdom, and Vashti ". . . calmly met her fate, And left the palace of the

King, Proud of her spotless name—A woman who could bend to grief but would not bend to shame" (p. 111).

Finally, another poem that might be used in a discussion of nurses as women and as professionals is "Woman" (Morrison, 1992). This short poem tells of a woman, who after thousands of insults and years of being passive, becomes Saint Joan, "a determined guerilla in the centuries-old, undeclared war against her" (p. 132). It might be used to initiate a discussion of the historical role of nurses as passive, dependent handmaidens, what nurses have done to fight against that kind of powerlessness, and what still needs to be done in order for nurses to be autonomous.

Film and Television

Philadelphia (1993), the award-winning film starring Tom Hanks and Denzel Washington, is the story of a young attorney who is diagnosed with AIDS and loses his job because of his illness. For use in a unit on professionalism, students might be asked to view the film from the perspective of a nurse who is the case manager for this individual, asking, for example, how she could serve as an advocate for him or what kind of support he needs to deal with his illness and its ramifications? The main character in this film also could be used to initiate a discussion of what it means to believe in something and fight for it, a concept that certainly fits with the study of professionalism.

Another popular film, *Top Gun* (1986), starring Tom Cruise, portrays a cocky jet fighter pilot who is out to prove something and be the very best. In the process he alienates himself from his peers and jeopardizes the success of his team's mission. When examining the idea of working as part of a team, faculty could use this film to illustrate the effect one member of the team can have on the overall outcome, if he is not really working as part of the group. Students could then be asked to do an analysis of a student group in which they might be involved, looking at how each individual—including themselves—contributes to or inhibits the progress of the group.

In 1988, a made-for-television movie, *Sentimental Women Need Not Apply*, was aired. This is an excellent historical account of nursing's history that incorporates photographs of past events, such as the Crimean and Civil Wars, clips from films about or involving nurses, and quotes from nursing leaders. It documents the relationship between social and political events and the development of the profession, and it shows how nurses truly led the way in so many areas of public health but never seized the power that could have accompanied those significant contributions. This documentary could be used to examine the interrelationship of social–political trends and nursing, nurse–physician relationships, nursing's image at the turn of the century and at present, and the success or failure of nurses to take responsibility for the development of the profession, one of the values of a professional noted earlier in this discussion.

More recent television programs also could be used to examine nursing's image. *ER, General Hospital, Chicago Hope,* and *Nightingales* (a show that was short-lived because nurses actively campaigned against it) all include a variety of nurse characters. Students might be assigned to view several episodes of one or more of these shows and describe the ways in which the nurses are portrayed, how they dress, and how they interact with patients, physicians, family members, and others, among other areas. Having students then discuss their analyses would probably help the group realize that different observers "see" different things in a situation, they assign different meaning to what they see, and they react differently. Students also might be asked to suggest how the image of the nurses in these shows could be enhanced.

Television also offers public service shows that have relevance to the study of professionalism. *Ethics in America* is a 9-part series, aired on PBS, that presents panels of attorneys, clergy, physicians, politicians, and others who struggle with ethical questions. In assigning students to view this series, or particular segments of it, faculty might ask some to describe the nature of the ethical dilemma itself and how it was resolved. Other students might be assigned to describe the dress, demeanor, articulateness, modes of interprofessional interaction, and professional demeanor exhibited by selected panel members. Still other students might be assigned to describe how the professional nurse was, could be, or should be integral to such interdisciplinary discussions.

The 1987 television production of "Baby Girl Scott," starring John Lithgow, also deals with ethical dilemmas, but portrays them through a very realistic story. The film tells of a premature infant's parents' fight for the right to have some say in treatment decisions for their child and the right to let the infant die. It can help students vicariously experience the traumas faced by the parents as well as the emotional challenges they and the health care professionals face in dealing with such situations. Students could be asked to reflect on the role of the professional nurse in these kinds of circumstances, how they could be patient/family advocates under conditions such as these, and what changes, if any, need to be made in the law and health care policy to minimize the trauma of these difficult decisions. Since this is a very powerful film that evokes strong emotions, faculty may need to give students adequate preparation for it, allow extended time for discussion, and be available to students should individuals wish to talk privately about their feelings.

Finally, the importance of living one's values is brought to light in the television series, *Due South*. This show is the story of a Royal Canadian Mounted Policeman who has been assigned to work with a police officer in Chicago. The "Mountie" has been reared to be totally honest and forthright, to treat all people with respect and dignity, and to follow the letter of the law. Working in an inner-city police precinct, alongside an officer who "bends the rules" as necessary, is a challenge to the "Mountie"'s principles, and he has to decide constantly where he will compromise and where not. As they watch this show, nursing students could consider their own values, to what extent and under what circumstances they have compromised or would be willing to compromise those values, what challenges they have faced or would expect to have to face in living up to their own standards when others around them are less committed, and how this kind of issue relates to one's development as a professional nurse.

Fine Arts

Drama

Mozart's final opera, *The Magic Flute* (1791), tells a story that includes religion, philosophy, a suicide attempt, male–female principles, class systems, value systems, and good versus evil forces of power. In this work, the noble Tamino seeks goodness and truth, while the lower-class Papageno seeks food, drink, and a pretty woman. After watching this childlike, fairy-tale opera, students could engage in a debate about male–female similarities and differences, the concept of androgyny, the ways in which each of us must integrate differences within ourselves, and the intrapersonal conflicts such integration often produces. As professional nurses, they will have to resolve such internal conflict; perhaps they could be asked to project how they might deal with such situations in the future.

Faust (1856), an opera by Verdi, is the story of an aging philosopher who is despondent and alone and resolves to end his life by taking poison. In his despair he invoks Satan, and Mephistopheles appears, promising youth and the sensual gratification Faust wants. In return, he requires that Faust sign a document promising his services in the nether regions. Faust signs the paper, enjoys the beauty of life for a short time, but that pleasure ends in tragedy, and he is as despondent as ever. This dramatic work presents an ethical dilemma not unlike dilemmas professional nurses face daily, namely, holding on to their values or "selling out" for some type of promise. Faculty might ask students to reflect on when they have held fast to the things they believe in, what difficulties that presents, the conditions that might make them give up what they value, and so on. Such reflection increases their awareness of their own values and the importance of knowing what it is that one does, indeed, believe.

Finally, the 1993 play, *Miss Evers' Boys* by David Feldshuh, is a dramatic representation of the effects of the Tuskegee syphilis study on the men who were subjects and the nurse who worked with them. Miss Evers recruited and cared for the poor, African American men who, for four decades, were studied by the government in an effort to prove that syphilis was a racially defined disease. Throughout the study—and in the interest of science—treatment that would have cured these men was withheld. This very moving play is an excellent example for use in a discussion of the ethics of research, as well as in an examination of the personal dilemmas Miss Evers and other nurses often face.

Music

There are many songs that deal with supporting another through difficult times, and these all could be used in a study of professionalism. In previous chapters, some of these songs were mentioned as ways to stimulate an understanding of the nurse-patient relationship. However, they also could be used in a discussion of nurse-nurse relationships. Any of the following songs would be good for this purpose: "Bridge Over Troubled Water" by Simon and Garfunkel, "He Ain't Heavy, He's My Brother" by Neil Diamond, "United We Stand" by The Brotherhood of Man, "Reach Out I'll Be There" by the Four Tops, and "Lean on Me" by Bill Withers. After listening to one or several of these pieces, students might be asked to read articles about nurses "eating their young," observe the interactions among nurses in the clinical areas where they affiliate, think about nurse-nurse support as a component of nursing's image, and compare nurse-nurse interactions to those observed between members of other professions. They then could propose strategies for how nurses could unite, how they could support their nursing colleagues in practice, and what nurses could do to present an image that is more collegial than confrontational.

Because learning about professionalism and how to be a professional must involve attention to one's own values if one is to succeed, songs that focus on personal challenges or strengths could be used in the educational process. "One Moment in Time" by Whitney Houston, inspired by Olympic athletes, deals with personal responsibility and holding oneself to high standards. Helen Reddy's ever popular "I Am Woman," tells of a woman who is wise, but gained that wisdom through struggling; again, the challenge of taking responsibility for one's life is evident in this song. Finally, "My Way," sung by Frank Sinatra is the story of a man who, as his life draws to a close, reflects on what he has done in life, the most important aspect of which was that he did it his way; this song conveys the message that we must be true to our values, make decisions for ourselves, and be accountable for the consequences of our actions.

"Nurses Change Lives"[2] is a song written and sung by Beth Reinhart, R. N. It relates how nurses change lives day after day and in so many ways: through teaching, caring, sharing, offering kindness, showing compassion, giving, listening, learning, and laughing. Students could be asked to verify if the roles of the nurse described in this song are congruent with their readings and what they have observed in practice. They also might be challenged to compose their own song—melody and lyrics, or lyrics only—that

---

2. This tape is available from Hart Songs, Inc., 2818 S.W. Indian Trail, Topeka, KS 66614.

conveys their insights about the role of the nurse and what it means to be a professional.

In the Broadway play *Miss Saigon* (1988) one of the Marines who had served there becomes involved with the well-being of the children of American servicemen and Vietnamese women. He sings an extremely poignant song, "Bui–Doi"—"the dust of life"—that could be used in nursing education. In this song, the Marine acknowledges that he thought he wouldn't give a damn about Vietnam after returning home, but then he saw a camp for children fathered by U.S. soldiers, and was haunted by their plight. The sight of so many innocent children abandoned in camps and shunned by their own countrymen as well as the United States reminded him of what we *failed* to do in Vietnam and how we often forget about or ignore those failures.

After faculty give students background information about the Vietnam war, the play, and the song, students could listen to the words and feelings expressed in it. They could then participate in a discussion about the responsibility nurses have for those who are underserved, ignored, alienated, and forgotten for whatever reason. Such an exercise may help students realize their social responsibility as professionals and speculate on how nurses could help these souls who need a chance to live a quality life.

Painting

"The Nanny" by Norman Rockwell is a humorous depiction of the frustrations that sometimes accompany caring for others. This painting shows a young woman, wearing a blue uniform with a white apron and white nurses' cap, sitting with her elbows on her knees, her chin held in her hands, and her eyes cast heavenward. Sitting at her side is a baby, crying hysterically, with his toys strewn about and his full bottle sitting untouched. Students might be asked to study the face of the nanny, list the emotions they think she might be experiencing in this situation, then interview their peers or nurses in the agencies where they affiliate about whether they ever experience such emotions and if so, under what circumstances. Such an exercise could help students realize that nurses are not always perfect "angels of mercy" who have no needs of their own. This realization could then be followed by a discussion of what nurses could do to prevent themselves from burning out or becoming so overwhelmed with the challenges of their role that they withdraw or fail to practice in a truly professional manner.

A well-known painting that conveys strength of personal convictions as well as physical labor is "American Gothic" by Grant Wood. This picture of an elderly man and woman, each holding a farm implement and looking straight ahead with somewhat stern expressions on their faces, suggests the difficult work they do on a daily basis as well as the commitment they have to a certain way of life. Students looking at this painting might be challenged to think about the physical or psychomotor abilities needed by a nurse in different settings or areas of practice and suggest ways they could maintain that kind of stamina. Discussions about the role of the professional nurse often fail to address the physical dimension, but this painting could be used to bring that element of practice to light.

"Florence Nightingale Receiving the Wounded at Scutari" by Jerry Barratt shows the founder of modern nursing at the hospital near the battle site where wounded soldiers are being brought. It depicts Nightingale's compassion and concern for the well-being of her patients, the adverse conditions they all faced, and the caring nurse-patient relationship. In addition to using this work as part of a discussion of nursing's history, it could serve as a stimulus for a discussion of making decisions in uncertainty, facilitating change, creating a positive environment for patients and fellow nurses, and dealing with crises and adversity. All of these are elements of the concept of professionalism, and all are issues that students need to address.

"Night Duty" by Franklin Boggs shows similar conditions but in a more recent situation. Here an army nurse is seen in a ward with several cots lined up next to each other; only sheer gauze separates the cots. The nurse is walking between the cots, holding a flashlight and checking on each patient. Again, this painting could be used during a discussion of the dedication, vigilance, compassion, and unending work required of professional nurses.

Finally, "The Nightingale Window" is a tribute to and glorification of nursing. It is a six-panel stained glass work designed by Reynolds, Francis, and Rohnstock in 1938 that hangs in the National Cathedral in Washington, DC. This piece of art reflects the dignity of nurses and of the profession, as well as the many ways in which nurses contribute to the well-being of others. As they examine the image of nurses and nursing, students might be directed to examine the panels in this window, describe the image that is portrayed, analyze how that image has changed in recent years and what has contributed to that change, and propose strategies to improve the current image.

Sculpture

Rodin's "The Thinker" conveys the notion of intellect and thoughtfulness, and "Moses" by Michelangelo seems to make a statement about wisdom. Both of these are characteristics of professional nurses, and both may be used to initiate or conclude a discussion of the need for ongoing education, how to take responsibility for maintaining and expanding one's knowledge base, whether there is a place in the clinical arena for making decisions based on wisdom and intuition, the need for nursing research, and how the public and other members of the health care team perceive the intellectual component of nursing practice.

A lasting tribute to all women who served in the military was dedicated in 1994 in Washington, DC. The "Vietnam Women's Memorial" depicts a nurse holding a wounded soldier in her arms while another looks skyward, anticipating a helicopter. Not only does the message of the monument itself have relevance in a discussion of professionalism; the story behind the creation and dedication of it also warrants discussion. Nurses were very instrumental in initiating the creation of this memorial, pursuing all the necessary approvals, and seeing it through to completion; as such, it serves as a testament to what nurses can do when there is a dedication to a goal or cause, and when one truly believes in something.

Finally, "The Spirit of Nursing" in Arlington Cemetery is a monument to nurses themselves. This tall, graceful statue of a nurse wearing a cape and gazing out over the rows of tombstones of nurses who served their country was created in 1938 by Frances Luther Rich. It is the only monument to commemorate military nurses, and gives one a sense of pride in the profession. Students might be asked to think about what it is about their work that gives them a sense of pride and accomplishment and what they do to acknowledge the contributions of their nursing peers. This kind of thoughtful reflection heightens students' awareness of their broad responsibility to the long-term health of the profession.

CONCLUSION

As is true for so many of the other concepts integral to nursing curricula, the concept of professionalism is multidimensional and complex. As a result, nurse educators are challenged to consider ways in which students could be helped to reflect on their personal and professional values, to utilize teaching and learning strategies that help students consider the meaning of their values in their lives as nurses, and to design learning experiences that make the many aspects of professionalism come alive for students. The examples from the arts and humanities provided here are but a sampling of how these goals could be achieved. It is hoped that such examples will help faculty be more creative in their teaching.

REFERENCES

American Nurses Association. (1976). *Code for nurses with interpretive statements*. Kansas City, MO: Author.

Anderson, P. (1985). *Children's hospital*. New York: Harper & Row.

Andreoli, K. G., Carollo, J. R., & Pottage, M. W. (1990). Marketing strategies: Projecting an image of nursing that reflects achievement. In E. C. Hein & M. J. Nicholson (Eds.), *Contemporary leadership behavior: Selected readings* (3rd ed., pp. 41–50). Glenview, IL: Scott, Foresman/Little, Brown.

Author Unknown. (1941). It can be done. In A.L. Alexander (Compiler), *Poems that touch the heart* (p.274). New York: Doubleday.

Bennis, W. (1989). *On becoming a leader*. Reading, MA: Addison–Wesley.

Bright, F. (1984). *Decisions*. New York: St. Martin's Press.

Brower, P. J. (1983). The power to see ourselves. In E. G. Collins (Ed.), *Executive success: Making it in management* (pp. 15–28). New York: Wiley.

Campbell, E. R. (1857). *The heroine of Scutari and other poems*. New York: Dana and Co.

Chandler, G. (1992). Nurses in the news: From invisible to visible. *Journal of Nursing Administration, 22*(2), 11–12.

Covey, S. R. (1989). *The 7 habits of highly effective people: Restoring the character ethic*. New York: Simon and Schuster.

Crichton, J. (1986). *Delivery: A nurse–midwife's story*. New York: Warner Books.

Curtin, L. L. (1985). Packing the professional for success. *Nursing Management, 16*(4), 7–8.

Dickens, C. (1910). *Martin Chuzzlewit.* New York: Macmillan.

Donahue, M. P. (1985). *Nursing: The finest art. An illustrated history.* St. Louis: Mosby.

Felleman, H. (Selected by). (1936). *The best loved poems of the American people.* Garden City: Doubleday & Co.

Flexner, A. (1915). Is social work a profession? *Proceedings of the National Conference of Charities and Correction.* Chicago: Hildman.

Frede, R. (1985). *The nurses.* Boston: Houghton Mifflin.

Fulghhum, R. (1986) *All I really need to know I learned in kindergarten.* New York: Ivy Books.

Gino, C. (1982). *The Nurse's Story.* New York: Bantam Books.

Harper, F. E. (1993). Vashti. In I. Linthwaite (Ed.), *Ain't I a woman!* (pp. 110–111). New York: Wing Books.

Hein, E. C., & Nicholson, M. J. (Eds.) (1990). *Contemporary leadership behavior: Selected readings* (3rd ed.). Glenview, IL: Scott, Foresman/Little, Brown.

Heron, E. (1987). *Intensive care: The story of a nurse.* New York: Ivy Books.

Hinshaw, A. S. (1990). Socialization and resocialization of nurses for professional nursing practice. In E. C. Hein & M. J. Nicholson (Eds.), *Contemporary leadership behavior: Selected readings* (3rd ed., pp. 17–32). Glenview, IL: Scott, Foresman/Little, Brown.

Holloway, E. (Ed.). (1932). *The uncollected poetry and prose of Walt Whitman* Vol. I. New York: Peter Smith.

James, P. D. (1971). *Shroud for a nightingale.* New York: Warner Books.

Jones, A. H. (Ed.). (1988). *Images of nurses: Perspectives from history, art, and literature.* Philadelphia: University of Pennsylvania Press.

Kalisch, B. J., & Kalisch, P. A. (1990). Improving the image of nursing. In E. C. Hein & M. J. Nicholson (Eds.), *Contemporary leadership behavior: Selected readings* (3rd ed., pp. 33–39). Glenview, IL: Scott, Foresman/Little, Brown.

Kilmer, J. (1919, August 29). In memoriam: Florence Nightingale. *New York Times,* 4.

Lindbergh, A. M. (1955). *Gift from the sea.* New York: Pantheon Books.

Lindbergh, A. M. (1956). Two citadels. In A. M. Lindbergh, *The unicorn and other poems* (p. 9). New York: Pantheon Books.

Linedecker, C. L. & Burt, W. A. (1990). *Nurses who kill.* New York: Windsor Publishing Co.

Malcolm, A. H. (1987). *This far and no more.* New York: Times Books.

Moloney, M. M. (1992). *Professionalization of nursing: Current issues and trends* (2nd ed.). Philadelphia: Lippincott.

Morrison, L. (1992). Woman. In S. H. Martz (Ed.), *If I had my life to live over I would pick more daisies* (p. 132). Watsonville, CA: Papier–Mache.

Palmer, M. (1982). *The sisterhood*. New York: Bantam Books.

Paul, S. (1991). Remodeling the image of nursing: A powerful strategy for clinical nurse specialists. *Clinical Nurse Specialist, 5*(3), 156–158.

Paulus, T. (1972). *Hope for the flowers*. New York: Paulist Press.

Porter, R. T., Porter, M. J., & Lower, M. S. (1990). Enhancing the image of nursing. In E. C. Hein & M. J. Nicholson (Eds.), *Contemporary leadership behavior: Selected readings* (3rd ed., pp. 51–57). Glenview, IL: Scott, Foresman/ Little, Brown.

Roberts, S. J. (1983). Oppressed group behavior: Implications for nursing. *Advances in Nursing Science, 5*(4), 21–30.

Shem, S. (1978). *The House of God*. New York: Dell Publishing Co.

Silverstein, S. (1981). "This bridge." In S. Silverstein, *A light in the attic* (p. 169). New York: HarperCollins Publishers.

Stafford, L. (1987). Creative image building for nurse managers. *Today's OR Nurse, 9*(1), 25–29.

Strasen, L. L. (1992). *The image of professional nursing: Strategies for action*. Philadelphia: Lippincott.

Taylor, E. R. (1972). *Welcome Eumenides*. New York: George Braziller.

Wagenknecht, E. (1986). *Henry Wadsworth Longfellow—His poetry and prose*. New York: Ungar.

Yura, H. (1989). Enhancing the image of the nurse: The role of the nurse supervisor. Part I. *Health Care Supervisor, 7*(2), 1–11.

Index

Abandon Ship (film), 137
Activity theory on aging, 65
Advertisements, communication
    techniques in, 223
Advocacy role of nurses, 259
   for aging population, 67
   for dying patients, 118
Aesop's fables, 241–242
Affective aspects. *See* Emotions
Affirmative action, compared to diversity,
    151–152
"After Death" (painting by Gericault),
    140
Aging, 7, 61–79
   biological theories on, 62–63, 64–65
   communication ability in, 215
   definition of, 62–63
   demographics of, 63
   developmental tasks in, 62
     in families, 169–173
   and diversity of age, 149
     resources on, 164
   dramas on, 76
   family functions in, 168, 169–173
   films and television programs on, 72–76
   literature on, 67, 68–72
   music on, 76–77
   nursing care in, 66–67
   paintings on, 77–78
   photography on, 78
   psychosocial theories on, 62, 65–66
AIDS
   dramas on, 139
   films on, 138, 276
   novels on, 180

   photography on, 206
   short stories on, 201
   television programs on, 205
All I Really Need to Know I Learned in
    Kindergarten (Fulghum), 271–272
Alzheimer's disease, 202
"American Gothic" (painting by Wood),
    281–282
Anatomy of an Illness (Cousins), 128
Andre's Mother (film), 138
Angels in America (drama), 139
Anonymity: The Secret Life of an American
    Family (Bergman), 180
Assessment process, 81–96
   caring in, 82–83
   on communication, 211, 219
   context of, 84–86
   definition of, 82–89
   films and television programs on,
     91–92
   informed approach to, 83–84
   literature on, 90–91
   paintings on, 92–93
   on personal strengths and weaknesses,
     261–262
   photography on, 93–94
   purposive nature of, 87–89
   reflection in, 86–87
   sculptures on, 94–95
Autonomy in professional nursing
    practice, 259

Baby Girl Scott (television program),
    277–278
Beaches (film), 111

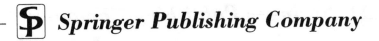

Springer Publishing Company

SPIRITUALITY IN NURSING
From Traditional to New Age

Barbara Stevens Barnum, RN, PhD, FAAN

In this thoughtful examination of
the reemergence of spirituality as
an important factor in nursing
practice, the author traces nursing's
involvement with spirituality from
its historical ties with religion to the
current interest in alternative health
methods. New nursing theories that
involve spirituality, such as those of
Dossey, Newman, and Watson are
described. And nursing trends are

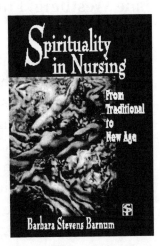

put in the larger context of trends in society and other
disciplines, such as psychology, physics, and philosophy.

Contents:

- Spirituality in Nursing: Origins, Development, Overview
- Spirituality and Nursing's History
- Spirituality as a Component in Nursing Theory
- Developmental Theories: Is There a Spiritual Phase?
- Spirituality and the Emerging Paradigm
- Nursing Theorists in the New Paradigm
- Nursing and Healing
- Spirituality and Ethics: A Contrast in Forms
- Ethics and Philosophy
- Spirituality and the Mind
- Spirituality, Disease, and Death
- Spirituality and Religion
- Spiritual Therapeutics

1995   176pp   0-8261-9180-0   hardcover

536 Broadway, New York, NY 10012-3955 • (212) 431-4370 • Fax (212) 941-7842

Ⓢ *Springer Publishing Company*

FOSTERING LEARNING IN SMALL GROUPS
A Practical Guide

Jane Westberg, PhD & Hilliard Jason, MD, EdD

Drawing on years of experience, the authors address the questions that educators may have about small group teaching in the health sciences. The first half of the book focuses on practical strategies involved in planning and facilitating learning in small groups. The authors discuss the characteristics of effective groups and emphasize the importance of using a collaborative approach. The second half focuses on planning for and leading small groups that have specific purposes such as providing a forum for discussion and dialogue, teaching communication skills, and helping learners reflect on their patient care experiences, and more. The book's broad orientation and practical emphasis will be useful to all educators in health care.

Contents:

- Generic Concepts and Issues
- The Role of Small Groups in Health Professions Education
- Preparing for Leading Small Groups
- Preparing Yourself for Leading Groups
- Leadership Tasks and Strategies During Group Sessions
- Co-leading Small Groups
- Planning for and Leading Groups with Specific Tasks
- Facilitating Discussions and Dialogues
- Doing Problem-Based Learning
- Teaching Communication Skills
- Processing Patient/Client Care and Other Experiences
- Providing Support to Learners

Springer Series on Medical Education
1996   310pp   0-8261-9330-7

536 Broadway, New York, NY 10012-3955 • (212) 431-4370 • Fax (212) 941-7842

𝕊 *Springer Publishing Company*

ADVANCING NURSING EDUCATION WORLDWIDE

Doris Modly, RN, PhD,
Renzo Zanotti, IP, AFD, Dott., PhD (C),
Piera Poletti, & **Joyce J. Fitzpatrick**,
RN, PhD, FAAN, Editors

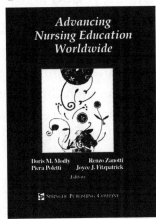

The contributors of this comprehensive book describe global trends in nursing education, share innovative approaches to it, report and develop cross-cultural and collaborative research, and provide a model for future international collaborations in nursing. The book concludes with a blueprint for action that nurses can apply to improve the status of nursing education.

Partial Contents:

Part I: Nursing Education Requirements Worldwide. Global Trends in Nursing Education: A World Health Organization Perspective, *J. Salvage* • Broadening Nursing Boundaries Through Nursing Education and Nursing Education Research, *R. Zanotti*

Part II: Teaching Practices Worldwide. Designing Curriculum to Advance Nursing Science and Professional Practice, *D.M. Modly*

Part III: Issues Important to Nurse Educators Worldwide. Management Education for Nurses in the United States, *S.A. Ryan & C. Conway-Welch* • Computers in Nursing Education, *M. Tallberg* • Re-entry of Students, *D. McGivern*

Part IV: Advancing Research in Nursing Education. Pathways to Implementing Nursing Education Research Globally, *J.J. Fitzpatrick* • A Blueprint for Advancing Nursing Education Research Globally, *Scientific Committee Members*

1995   200pp   0-8261-8650-5   hardcover

536 Broadway, New York, NY 10012 • (212) 431-4370 • Fax (212) 941-7842

$\boxed{\textbf{SP}}$ *Springer Publishing Company*

INCREASING PATIENT SATISFACTION
A Guide for Nurses

Roberta L. Messner, RNC, PhD, CPHQ
Susan J. Lewis, RN, PhD, CS

This manual guides nurses and others in the health care setting through the fundamentals of ensuring a satisfied "customer." It illustrates the many components of quality care, including how to provide clear and adequate information, create a hospitable environment, handle complaints efficiently, and design and utilize surveys of client satisfaction.

The authors draw from the principles of continuous quality improvement and other lessons learned from the business world, in addition to nursing's rich tradition of service. Written with warmth, sensitivity, and clarity, the book is an excellent resource for nursing students and practicing nurses. Health care institutions seeking good client relations will find this a suitable text for in-service training.

Contents:

What Do Patients Really Want? • The Changing American Healthcare Scene and Patient Satisfaction• Quality Isn't a Coincidence• Yes, Patients Do Have Rights • Patient Education: A Key to Increased Satisfaction • Creating a Hospitable and Healing Environment • How to Handle a Customer Complaint • Looking for the Lesson: Measuring/Evaluating Patient Satisfaction Findings • Be Kind to Yourself and Your Coworkers: A Plan for Enhanced Morale and Patient Satisfaction

1996   240pp   0-8261-9250-5   hardcover

536 Broadway, New York, NY 10012-3955 • (212) 431-4370 • Fax (212) 941-7842